T0366901

Sensory Processing
Challenges

SENSORY
PROCESSING
CHALLENGES

Effective Clinical Work
with Kids & Teens

LINDSEY BIEL

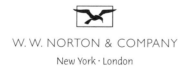

W. W. NORTON & COMPANY
New York · London

For information about permission to reproduce selections from this book, write to
Permissions, W. W. Norton & Company, Inc., 500 Fifth Avenue, New York, NY 10110

For information about special discounts for bulk purchases, please contact
W. W. Norton Special Sales at specialsales@wwnorton.com or 800-233-4830

Manufacturing by Quad Graphics, Fairfield
Book design by Tom Ernst
Production manager: Leeann Graham

Library of Congress Cataloging-in-Publication Data

Biel, Lindsey.
Sensory processing challenges : effective clinical work with
kids & teens / Lindsey Biel. — First edition.
pages cm. — (A Norton professional book)
Includes bibliographical references and index.
ISBN 978-0-393-70834-9 (hardcover)
1. Sensory integration dysfunction in children.
2. Sensory disorders in children—Treatment. I. Title.
RJ496.S44B54 2014
618.92'8—dc23
2013041179

ISBN: 978-0-393-70834-9

W. W. Norton & Company, Inc., 500 Fifth Avenue, New York, N.Y. 10110
www.wwnorton.com

W. W. Norton & Company Ltd., Castle House, 75/76 Wells Street, London W1T 3QT

1 2 3 4 5 6 7 8 9 0

This book is dedicated
to my clients, who amaze me
each and every day.

CONTENTS

ACKNOWLEDGMENTS

What you focus on expands. As an occupational therapist, the focus of my work has always been to optimize my clients' strengths in order to help them overcome their challenges. At the same time, I have had the great fortune of wonderful people in my life who help keep me strong.

I owe a lifetime of loving thanks to my mother, who was so encouraging about this project and who, when I felt as if I were juggling sea otters while attempting to balance writing this book, treating my caseload of kids and teens, teaching workshops across the country, and having a personal life, simply said, "I know you can do it." As usual, she was right. Thanks as well to my beloved brothers, Timothy and Michael, and my sister, Laura, all of whose love and support have always meant so much to me. Knowing how proud our father would have been means so much too. And having you out there rocking the planet, Johnny B. Azari, makes the world a better place.

I am greatly indebted to Andrea Costella Dawson, my thoughtful, gentle, and inspiring editor at W. W. Norton, who approached me with this book idea. As I stood by the iconic New York Public Library lions across the street from her office after our first meeting, my heart and mind raced with excitement about the impact this book could make in the lives of children and their families. Sophie Hagen, assistant managing editor of Norton Professional Books, and copyeditor Karen Fisher did superb jobs transforming my manuscript into an actual book.

I am deeply grateful to photographer Timothy Archibald, whose exceptional image of his extraordinary son Eli graces the cover of this book. My autographed copy of his book, *Echolilia*, is a truly prized possession.

Special thanks go to occupational therapist Dr. Tina Champagne for her wisdom and guidance; nutritionist Kelly Dorfman who knows so much; speech language pathologists Melissa Wexler Gurfein and Melanie Potock; developmental optometrist Dr. Fran Reinstein; audiologist Louise Levy; physical therapist Kelly Sindle; and occupational therapists Markus Jarrow and Huck Ho for their encouragement, support, and generosity. Heartfelt thanks go to Julie Bagley, Ida Zelaya, Melissa Zacherl, Susan Dolin Rothschild, Molly Kiely, Chantal Sicile-Kira, Suzanne Peters, Cecilia Cruse, Jennifer Mitchell, Jenny Davis, and Lisa Witt as well, for their invaluable help. A round of enthusiastic (but not *too* loud) applause goes to autism advocates Chloe Rothschild and Jeremy Sicile-Kira for sharing their stories, as well as to Joanne and Victoria Sciortino, Bryan, Erin, and others who wished to remain anonymous. May the challenges you've shared help to smooth the path for others.

Temple Grandin's enthusiasm for the practical strategies in this book means so much to me. I am deeply honored by her support and encouragement.

Boundless thanks to Rick Frankel for technical support and so much more. I joked that I would write this book despite you, but really, I could not have done it without you.

Finally, this book could never have been written without my sensitive, sweet, smart, and funny clients and their families. You teach me, you inspire me, you make me strong.

INTRODUCTION

Robin can't sit still. She is always fidgeting with something, chewing on her shirtsleeves, getting up from the table. What's going on?

Max is smart and interested in learning, but he refuses to follow classroom routines and is sometimes aggressive with classmates in the halls and at recess. What's going on?

Lily wakes up every night crying inconsolably and is comforted only when her parents let her sleep in their room. What's going on?

James loves lining up toys, hums continuously, hates getting messy, and has a meltdown when there is an unexpected change in routine. What's going on?

What is going on indeed? The kids we work with are marvelously complex and sometimes baffling. Robin is always on the go, to the point that it is becoming a real bother to her parents, teachers, and peers. Is it due to attention-deficit/hyperactivity disorder (ADHD) or something else? Why is Max so avoidant and aggressive? Does Lily have an emotional or behavioral problem or is something bothering her body? Are James's behaviors purely symptoms of autism or might it be something else?

This book will help you consider the role sensory processing difficulties may play—and give you tools and strategies to help. Robin may be able to focus better if given acceptable ways to obtain movement and touch input. Max might be able to handle the noise and chaos of a busy classroom or playground if given ear protection for his oversensitive ears and simple classroom accommodations. Lily might sleep better if given a bedtime routine that starts with a deep-pressure massage and ends with all lights off and a white noise machine turned on. James may begin to let go of his controlling and self-stimulatory behaviors as he feels less at the mercy of overwhelming sensory stimulation he cannot control.

To fully understand a child's world, clinicians must consider how a child experiences the nonstop stream of sensory input coming from the external environment as well as from inside his own body. These sensory experiences shape everything children, from toddlers to teens, do and feel.

Fact is, children first learn about and understand the world through their senses. Sensory processing is how their brains interpret the feel, sounds, tastes, sights, and smells of things that are constantly being sensed from both inside and outside their bodies. The senses include familiar ones—touch, vision, sound, taste, and smell—and some that are less well known. The vestibular sense relies on receptors in the inner ear to tell us about movement and gravity. The proprioceptive sense uses input from joints, muscles, and connective tissue to tell us where our body parts are in space. These sensory modalities integrate seamlessly and automatically to provide us with an accurate, reliable picture of the world and our place in it, enabling us to behave and respond accordingly.

People with sensory processing challenges are wired differently. Some of the streams of sensory input are disrupted, and some of the senses do not link up well in the brain. As a result, people with sensory problems do not always have dependable, consistent sensory information to work with, making it difficult to interpret and respond adaptively to everyday life experiences. You'll read about some of the research showing neurobiological differences in children with sensory processing difficulties in Chapter 3.

It is essential for mental health clinicians and others who work with and care about children—and adults, for that matter—to take such sensory differences into account. Challenges with sensory processing significantly impact behavior and function, shaping our experiences, feelings, and actions throughout the day—while learning at school, playing and socializing, building motor skills, developing self-esteem, and cultivating other core elements of ourselves.

Sensory processing challenges can range from quirky preferences and intolerances to sensory jumbling and extreme pain. Sensory issues cast a wide net, affecting kids, teens, and adults with diagnoses such as autism, ADHD, anxiety and mood disorders, and developmental delays as well as those who are otherwise neurotypical.

Many children with mild sensory issues do grow out of it, especially given compassionate guidance. For those with more significant difficulties, untreated sensory issues increasingly interfere with playing, learning, socializing, and developing a sense of self. For example, the child who is hypersensitive to touch and sound may become alienated and hypervigilant, showing classic fight-or-flight stress responses, avoiding people and situations perceived as intolerable or dangerous. The hyposensitive child may be hard to reach, chronically underaroused, inattentive, and lethargic. Whether a client is hyper- or hyposensitive to particular types of sensory input or struggles to process multisensory input simultaneously and regardless of any other diagnoses, assessing and addressing any sensory processing deficits should be an essential part of any treatment plan.

One of the great challenges of being a clinician—or parent or teacher for that matter—is knowing when to push a child forward, when to back off and try another day, and how often, and to what extent, to accommodate issues by modifying the environment or what the child is asked to do. When a person feels physically or emotionally uncomfortable or in pain due to sensory issues, he cannot function at his best. Yes, we do want him to be able to tolerate all kinds of experiences eventually. Yes, we do want to avoid situations that he is currently unable to tolerate. And yes, it's a good idea to accommodate sensitivities so he can function at his best right now.

I wrote *Raising a Sensory Smart Child: The Definitive Handbook for Helping Your Child With Sensory Processing Issues* along with the mother of a child I used to treat, to help parents, teachers, therapists, and other caregivers to develop the "sensory smarts" that enable the children they raise, teach, and love to flourish at home, at school, and in the community. Since then I have worked with hundreds of young children and teenagers along with their parents, teachers, and other therapists and have spoken to thousands of people at my workshops and online. Over and over, parents have voiced their frustration at having their child's problems misunderstood and often misidentified as well as their enormous relief about finally finding clinicians who understand sensory challenges and are ready and able to help.

Now I am delighted to present you with *Sensory Processing Challenges: Effective Clinical Work With Kids & Teens*, written to give clinicians in mental health and other disciplines who work with children the insights, information, and practical strategies needed to better understand and help kids, teens, and their families with a wide range of sensory processing issues.

Part I provides the nuts and bolts: a breakdown of all our sensory systems, how they look when they function well, and what happens when they don't. You will learn how to recognize sensory problems in clients and understand underlying issues and coexisting conditions. Part II guides you through the interventions: how to develop a therapeutic program for kids and teens facing sensory challenges; how to work with occupational therapists and other experts in the field to give your clients the best care possible; how to work compassionately with concerned parents; and finally, how to work respectfully and effectively with schools, a key component of a child's path to success.

I sincerely hope this book will give you the sensory strategies that will make a huge, lasting difference in the lives of the children and families you work with and care about.

Sensory Processing
Challenges

Part I

Recognizing Sensory Processing Challenges

CHAPTER 1

Your Client's Sensory World

Martin is a preschooler who rocks in his chair, puts things in his mouth, lines up toys, and plays by himself on the sidelines at recess, frequently flapping his hands at his sides. When his teacher or classmates speak to him, he doesn't seem to hear them and avoids eye contact. At home, he is content for hours building complex Lego structures. He typically becomes enraged when told to stop building and come to dinner, take a bath, or go to bed.

Jaden wanders around his kindergarten classroom, fidgeting with his clothing, kicking off his shoes, pulling books and supplies off shelves, and bumping into tables and classmates. During circle time, he calls out inappropriately and moves constantly, changing from cross-legged to kneeling to lying down. He virtually never sits still at school. At home he plays video games for hours. He is so exhausted by the end of the day that he sometimes puts himself to bed early.

Isabella is a teenager who does well academically but doesn't fit in at school. Her parents are fed up with arguing with her in the morning and let her wear whatever she wants. In the middle of winter she wears sandals and short-sleeved dresses with no tights. She sits alone and eats peanut butter and jelly sandwiches every day for lunch. The other kids think she's an oddball and have begun to avoid her. She seems anxious all the time. Her parents and teacher increasingly feel like they are walking on eggshells around her. It's getting harder and harder to tell

when she is going to have a meltdown about her homework or comply-
ing with what seems like a simple request.

At first glance, these lovely children seem to have fairly clear-cut
diagnoses. The preschooler shows signs of autism; the kindergartener
shows signs of ADHD; and the teenager may well have an anxiety
disorder. But is anything else going on? Why does Martin engage in
so many rigid, self-stimulatory behaviors? Is there something beneath
Jaden's continuous, impulsive motor activity? Why won't Isabella
dress and eat like her peers? Are some unrecognized sensory factors
interfering with the development of these children?

And what about the child who presents in the mental health clinic
in the throes of a manic state or in active psychosis? Can changing
that child's sensory state—his most primal, immediate experience of
the world—help him recover and return to baseline more quickly?

The children we work with and care about are incredibly complex
and the answers are rarely simple. In order to help, we have to navigate through the ambiguity of human existence and consider people
in their entirety, including how they experience everyday life through
their sensory systems.

WE FIRST LEARN THROUGH THE SENSES

All of us initially learn about the world and ourselves through our
senses. Starting in the womb, the fetus hears his mother's steady,
rhythmic heartbeat and the muffled sounds of the outside world. The
fetus bathes in warm amniotic fluid which provides hydrostatic compression against the skin, muscles, and connective tissue. He hears
sounds such as Mom's heartbeat and the blood whooshing through her
body as well as muffled sounds from the outside world. He startles
and his heart rate increases at loud, unexpected noise but slows down
when he hears his mother's voice. He figures out how to move around
inside that small, safe space as the nervous and musculoskeletal systems develop. All of these familiar sensory experiences in the womb
are replaced by new, stimulating movements, sounds, sights, touches,
and more once the baby is born. And so begins a lifetime of discovery.

The newborn is already a fully sensory being. He learns how to move his arms and hands, legs and feet, head and neck and torso. He increasingly mouths things and touches himself, others, and objects and discovers that people and things have a texture, temperature, and pliability. He hears sounds and orients his body to look toward the source, eventually sorting out those sounds into words, music, and ambient noise. His vision becomes more acute and he can focus on his hands and watch his parents move around.

He learns how to roll over, push up, and stay upright against the pull of gravity. He learns that everything has some kind of smell and taste, mouthing and smelling the source of nourishment whether bottle or breast, playing with his own fingers and feet and then toys and teethers. He learns to make his body parts work together to physically interact with toys and people. As he pulls in and sifts through hundreds of thousands of bits of sensory messages from within his own body and from the outside world, he begins to make sense of himself in relationship with other people and the environment.

Thus sensory information forms the foundation for all of life's lessons.

To reiterate the definition from the introduction, sensory processing is the way we transform the nonstop stream of sensory information entering our bodies—coupled with internal sensations—into meaningful messages. These sensory messages must register accurately on sensory receptors, travel smoothly up to the brain, and integrate with sensory information from other systems. For example, auditory receptors pick up sound waves and convert them into messages that travel to the auditory cortex of the brain. At the same time, vision receptors pick up changes in light, color, and movement and convert them into messages that travel to the visual cortex of the brain. These two streams of information integrate so that a child sees and hears a person, which in turn activates the vestibular (movement) system so that she can turn her head to get a better look at what's going on nearby. Smell receptors pick up a scent. All of this sensory input, taken together, generates a magnificent realization: It is Mommy! This neurological process happens automatically, continuously, and with astonishing accuracy for most people.

As the child develops, the ability to respond to these sensory messages increases. He learns he can touch that colorful bunny toy across the room if he crawls toward it. When a parent rocks him, he learns it is he that's moving and not the entire world. That dog walking toward him with a wagging tail is just saying hello, so he doesn't have to be afraid and cry. The vacuum cleaner is noisy but it won't hurt him. Broccoli is yummy, not yucky just because it's green.

As a child matures, she continues to explore the world through the senses and further refine her interactions. She challenges her sensory systems by trying new foods, learning to ride a bicycle, climbing trees, and visiting new places like zoos and amusement parks with different sights, sounds, smells, and movement experiences. She learns to suppress her innate need to move and explore in order to stay still and tune in with her eyes and ears, especially at school.

Adolescents and young adults, by now well accustomed to the sensuality of the everyday world, may ramp up sensory exploration, identifying comfort zones and testing limits by seeking out more intense sensory experiences such as listening to loud music, driving fast, experimenting with alcohol and drugs, and exploring sexual relationships.

Let's step back and look at what the sensory systems are all about.

MAKING SENSE OF SENSORY MODALITIES

We've all heard of the five basic senses: touch, sound, sight, taste, and smell. These are the senses that pick up detailed messages from the environment. There are additional senses that pick up information from within our own bodies too. These internal senses—proprioceptive, vestibular, and interoceptive—play an essential role in informing us about who we are and how we are. Working together, these senses integrate seamlessly to tell us what is going on around us and what we should do at any given time, giving us an accurate, reliable sense of ourselves and our place in the world.

Since no two people are alike, how we perceive and use sensory input varies. One person might perceive riding on a roller coaster as incredibly fun while another abhors it. One person may enjoy a fast-paced movie with lots of action-packed, colorful scenes and intense music while it makes another person's head spin. These differences are part of our unique personalities.

To fully understand variations in how different people react to sensory input, it's important to take a closer look at each sensory system.

Touch Sense

Our sense of touch—the tactile system—is the first sensory system to develop and our most primal means of comfort and self-knowledge. It is the largest sensory organ in the body, with several kinds of tactile receptors on the multiple layers of the skin and also lining the mouth, throat, digestive system, ears, genital openings, and other body parts.

It is through touching that a baby learns where her skin-covered body ends and the outside world begins. She learns she is safe and loved through cuddles, kisses, and touches all over as well as by being surrounded by soft toys and materials. As the child experiences less pleasant tactile input such as scratchy fabrics and rough splintery surfaces, she refines her perception of what feels good and what to avoid.

Touch is so much more than feeling caresses, furry animals, or a well-worn bathrobe. The tactile system includes several different experiences:

- Light touch is sensed by the movement of hair and the outer skin. Light touch experiences include feeling wind on exposed skin, casually brushing against someone, having your hair tousled, the movement of loosely fitting clothing, getting splashed with water or having sand on your body at the beach, walking through grass with bare feet, and so on. Light touch experiences tend to trigger alarm responses when they are unexpected. For example, if a mosquito lands on you, you swat it away, hopefully before you get bitten.

- Deep pressure is sensed by deeper skin layers when skin is compressed. Deep pressure includes bear hugs, massage, pushing against something, and so on. It tends to be relaxing as long as the pressure is distributed evenly over larger parts of the body that have thick skin and muscles. For example, a deep-pressure massage with broad, firm strokes on your back and shoulders feels wonderful, while something jabbing into your ribs feels terrible.

- Vibration consists of rhythmic tactile input and is usually very pleasant. Vibration experiences include using a vibrating tooth-brush, sitting on a vibrating chair at the nail salon, and leaning against a washing machine. For some, vibration is uniquely sooth-ing; some people fall asleep immediately in a car on the highway, for example. For people who do not enjoy vibration, sleeping on an airplane may be absolutely impossible.

- Temperature is perceived by thermoreceptors on the skin, in skel-etal muscles, and elsewhere in the body. Temperature preferences are subjective. One person may always be cold, wearing sweaters even in summer, while another person can't sleep under a blanket because she is always so hot.

- Pain sensations are sensed by specialized receptors on the skin, muscles, joints, and viscera called nociceptors, which alert the brain to physical damage. Pain sensations range from the mild though annoying pain of a paper cut or torn cuticle to the more intense pain of a severe headache or broken bone. Tolerance for pain varies. Some people are quite sensitive to what seems like a minor scrape while others can tolerate a great deal more pain before becoming distressed.

Tactile input falls into two categories—protective and discriminative—and each type of touch input travels to the brain along separate nerve pathways:

- Sensations such as temperature, pain, and light touch travel along neuroprotective pathways that help keep the body safe from harm. When you become too hot at the beach, you get under an umbrella or go indoors, hopefully before you get a sunburn. If you are cold, you put on a sweater or turn up the heat to help regulate your body temperature. If you get hurt, you try to remove yourself from the source of pain, take a painkiller, or get help.

- Discriminative touch runs along discriminative nerve tracts telling you the difference between things without seeing them. Discrimi-native touch lets you reach into a handbag and select a pen rather than a pencil. It also helps you localize touch experiences so you can pinpoint where that mosquito bit you without seeing the welt.

Most people adapt to sustained tactile input fairly quickly. Imagine yourself getting dressed in the morning. As you add each layer of clothing, you probably forget about it immediately. Another person may remain aware of the seams or clothing tags throughout the day. Likewise, it may take a few days or even weeks to adjust to changes in climate. Let's say you fly from Chicago to the Caribbean in midwinter. While some people will happily strip off layers of clothing and joyfully plunge into the ocean, others may struggle with the heat and humidity for hours or even days.

As you think about your client's tactile processing skills, consider habits and experiences such as these:

- Physical contact with loved ones as well as with casual acquaintances and total strangers.
- Comfort level with clothing and footwear, sleepwear, and bedding.
- Self-care tasks such as washing face and hair, brushing teeth, and trimming fingernails.
- Textures such as lotion, glue, or paint as well as foods that are slippery, crumbly, hard, mushy, and so on.
- Ability to adapt to changes in room and outdoor temperature, especially as seasons change.
- Ability to deal with pain ranging from headaches to menstrual cramps to broken bones and other medical issues.

Sound Sense

Dealing with sound is a complex, wonderful ability that begins with hearing muted noise in the womb and gets refined as we mature and learn to listen actively. We become increasingly sophisticated at auditory multitasking: We learn to block out street traffic while chatting with a friend and to recognize our own child's cry in a busy playground.

The auditory system includes both passive hearing and active listening. If anatomical structures are in good working order—that is, there is no hearing loss—hearing is an effortless process in which sound waves enter the ear and get converted into acoustic signals that travel to the brain. In contrast, listening requires some effort. Our ears pull in all kinds of noise, from the hum of electrical appliances to the roar of traffic to the specialized sounds of speech. In order to listen, we need to sort through this sound field, differentiate between sounds, and decide which to ignore and which to focus on. Auditory processing refers to how the central nervous system makes sense of all these sounds. It lets us tune out background noise and tune in the teacher's voice. It helps us hear the difference between closely related sounds such as *bad* and *pad* or *make* and *snake*.

Auditory processing has many components:

- Volume. Most of us detect sound at 0–15 decibels of volume. We all have our own comfort levels for volume, but there is general agreement when sounds are too loud. People with supersensitive hearing, also called hyperacusis, are able to hear things that most of us do not hear. For them, what seems like normal volume may be perceived as much too loud.

- Frequency refers to the number of sound waves per second. Higher-frequency sounds include high-pitched voices, whistles, hair dryers, and trumpets. Lower-frequency sounds include deep voices, idling trucks, vacuum cleaners, and air conditioners. Some people are more sensitive to certain sound frequencies, especially as very young children, though we become used to such sounds during typical development. Further, as we age, many of us lose our ability to hear certain frequencies, especially if we have listened to a lot of loud music or used power tools without adequate ear protection over the years.

- Auditory sensitivity. Most infants are quite sensitive to sound and do best in quiet, calm environments, though some seem to sleep "like a baby" no matter what clatter is going on. As a child develops, he adjusts to a variety of sounds, volume levels, and frequencies and responds to them in proportion to their sensory challenge, that is, without having a fight-or-flight stress response. While no one enjoys hearing a shrill fire alarm, most children are able to tolerate the noise—perhaps covering their ears—and get themselves rapidly to safety.

- Duration refers to how long sounds last. When learning a new language, it's much easier to decipher words when they are spoken slowly, with each sound elongated to allow the learner to truly hear them. In the same vein, if you are cooking and your oversensitive smoke alarm goes off briefly, you'll be fine. But if it blares on and on, the noise becomes increasingly distressing and intolerable.

- Localization refers to where a sound is coming from and helps us know where we are in space relative to others in the environment. When a baby hears the sound of her mother's voice, she turns and crawls toward her. When we hear an airplane zooming past, we know it is located in the sky and can hear it move toward our personal sound field and then away from it.

- Sound discrimination. From the moment he is born, and perhaps even in the womb, a child is learning to discriminate phonemes—the small sound units of speech. As he discriminates between each phoneme, differentiating between *cat* and *car*, *wake* and *wait*, and so on, he learns how sounds are strung together in certain patterns with specific patterns and rhythms and also learns to derive meaning based on tone of voice.

- Auditory filtering. As she develops, a child learns to ignore irrelevant sounds in the environment such as the refrigerator humming and to selectively focus her attention on what's important, such as her mother speaking. As she matures, she can increasingly sustain her concentration despite auditory distractions. The child begins to consciously tune out sounds from outside or the next room when her teacher is speaking in order to follow what is being said. In the cafeteria, a child learns how to chat with his friend despite loud, harsh echoes in a cavernous room.

In order to effectively process sound input, a person needs to be able to combine all of these auditory components to make logical emotional, intellectual, and behavioral connections. When you are driving and hear an ambulance siren, for example, you need to stay calm, quickly determine from which direction it is coming, and move out of the way.

As you think about your client's auditory processing skills, consider these factors:

- History of ear infections and respiratory illnesses.
- Ability to understand speech (receptive language); to express needs, wants, and ideas (expressive language); and understand the social dimensions of language (pragmatic language).
- Whether the person's voice is unusually loud or quiet.

- Any unusual reactions to loud, unexpected, and unusual noises.
- Ability to focus despite noise in the classroom, playground, and elsewhere.
- Ability to follow verbal directions.
- Socialization and friendship with peers.

Vision Sense

When we think of vision, we conjure up images such as gazing at a loved one, viewing a beautiful landscape, or reading a book. When we think of visual problems, we think of needing eyeglasses or even blindness. In actuality, the visual system is much more complex than whether or not our eyeballs see well. The eyes play a key role, of course, but what the brain does with visual input is what really counts. Not only do your eyes need to have good visual acuity (or be optically corrected via lenses), they also need to work together. It's just like a pair of binoculars: Each barrel carries its own visual information, yet they merge seamlessly into one image. Indeed, some people can see well through binoculars only if they close one eye (resulting in monocular, one-barrel vision). In the same way, some people cannot see 3-D movies well since they are unable to merge the two slightly different visual fields that generate the illusion of depth.

Functional Visual Processing

Your eyes pick up images of objects and people and this information travels to the brain to be processed for meaning: Is the visual stimulus novel or familiar? Important or irrelevant? Something that needs to be responded to or ignored?

As you walk down the sidewalk and see a car coming toward you on the road, your eye's sensor—the retina—picks up and encodes bits of data on rod (black-and-white sensors) and cone (color sensors) cells and sends signals to the brain to be matched up to prior experiences along with their emotional tags. You recognize that the car on the road moving at normal speed is innocuous visual information and block it out of immediate consciousness. If the car suddenly veers toward the curb, active awareness kicks in so you can analyze whether there is imminent danger. If so, all of your sensory systems engage to help you move quickly to safety.

A baby begins developing visual representations of the world by examining her hands and her parents' faces. She learns to look for the source of a sound. She learns to follow people as they move around the room. Her brain and eyes work together so she learns visual perspective: that the person who seems tiny far away is the same creature who looks big close up. She learns where her body is in space and in relation to objects as she reaches toward toys and food sources. She learns to keep the visual field stable so the room does not appear to move when she is moved through space. She learns to follow the trajectory of a moving ball in order to catch it. She develops a strong visual memory, remembering shapes and colors and the sequence of how letters are formed, and eventually how to read.

Some key visual processing skills include the following:

- Binocular vision refers to the ability of the eyes to work together to keep the visual field clear, with each object appearing as a single item with clearly defined edges. Difficulties with binocularity result in blurred images, eyestrain, and sometimes double vision, making it hard to learn to read, navigate through space, maintain eye contact with other people, sustain visual attention, and develop skills requiring eye-hand coordination such as learning to write and use scissors.

- Stereoscopic vision is the ability of the brain to combine the two slightly different images in each eye. This visual skill is essential to depth perception. Without stereoscopic vision, the world appears in flattened 2-D, making it hard to do things like climb stairs, identify how close people and objects are, tell when a ball is coming toward you in order to catch it, and so on.

- Ocular motor skills. In addition to keeping the visual field in focus, the muscles controlling the eyes are responsible for activities that require visual precision. Examples include following a moving object such as a softball flying through the air or friends running on the playground; fixating on an object as you move, such as keeping an eye on a basketball hoop as you dribble the ball toward it; smooth, sequenced scanning, such as reading lines of print in a book; and changing focus from one point to another, such as looking up at the teacher, looking down at the tabletop in order to write notes, and looking up again.

- Visual attention and visual memory. Children quickly learn to visually attend to items for longer periods and to analyze the salient details that enable the brain to store the visual information with increasing sophistication, especially as language develops. Very young children may lump all small animals into one category, so that both cats and dogs are doggies. As they learn to look for distinct features such as pointy ears, triangular noses, sizes, and different kinds of fur, they are able to differentiate between tabby cats, Maine coon cats, miniature and standard poodles, and golden and Labrador retrievers. The toddler who calls every crayon "blue" will soon be able to name a wide range of colors as she attends visually and learns the corresponding label. Ideally, the ability to sustain visual focus attention and build visual and auditory memory increases throughout the early school years.

- Visual-perceptual skills include figure-ground discrimination (ability to find a favorite book on a bookshelf), visual closure (ability to recognize an object without seeing the whole image, such as recognizing a toy truck when just part of a wheel is jutting out of a toy box), and form constancy (ability to perceive things as the same even if they differ in terms of context, size, position, or other variable; e.g., number 3 is always a 3 whether it is tiny, pink, upside down, or in a strange typeface).

As you think about your client's visual processing skills, consider these factors:

- Ability to see things nearby as well as far away.
- Complaints of tiredness, headaches, dizziness, or nausea.
- If the person squints, rubs, or opens and closes her eyes frequently.
- Tilts head to one side or closes one eye when looking at something or reading.
- Ability to concentrate for age-appropriate duration.
- Ability to block out extraneous people, objects, and movement in the periphery.
- Comfort in sunlight, glare, darkness, or under fluorescent and downcast light.

- Eye-hand coordination tasks such as catching a ball, throwing, stringing beads, cutting with scissors.
- Age appropriateness of reading skills.

Taste and Smell Senses

There's nothing like the lush fragrance of roses in full bloom, the aroma of cookies baking in the oven, the rich taste of a great, full-bodied red wine, or the yumminess of macaroni and cheese or whatever food you most enjoy.

Taste and smell sensations are intimately connected, providing us with some of the greatest pleasures in life while keeping our bodies safe. Our keen noses can detect up to 10,000 odors, including the stench of spoiled milk, stinky fish, and many (but not all) noxious gases. In contrast, only five tastes are picked up chemically by the tongue: salty, sweet, sour, bitter, and umami. Umami is the savory flavor of glutamic acid, which is present in foods such as cheese and soy sauce and is sometimes added to foods to enhance flavor in its salt form, monosodium glutamate (MSG).

Let's say you are given a slice of dill pickle with your eyes closed. Your tongue's taste buds pick up sourness; your tongue's tactile receptors pick up the smooth coolness and round shape; and your nose picks up the distinctive brininess and dill seasoning. Aha! It's a pickle. Your nose plays a major role in food enjoyment. If you have a head cold with nasal congestion, food will lack flavor and your appetite may be reduced.

When most people think about tasting food, they think about the tongue. However, flavor is a combination of taste on the tongue, smell in the nostrils, texture on the skin, and other sensory features such as temperature. While all taste buds have receptors for all tastes, you actually detect sweet best on the tip of your tongue, salty on the sides and tip, sour on the midsection and sides, and bitter toward the back. Meanwhile your nose is detecting the nuances that give foods their distinctive flavor. If you're not quite sure what the food is or whether you'll like it, you sniff a bit more before ingesting it. In order to really taste something, you need to dissolve it in saliva so your mouth waters when you start to eat or even smell something you like. As the food moves along your tongue surface, you pick up information about whether it is dry and crumbly, slippery, mushy, warm, cold, and so on. You chew it up and form it into the round mass called a bolus needed to swallow. And assuming you've formed your bolus and moistened up the works well, you swallow and prepare for more.

Smell and taste development begins in the womb. The smell of the amniotic fluid helps the fetus to develop a sense of smell and taste before she is even born. An infant will move away from nasty smells such as rotten eggs and smile at pleasant odors such as bananas. Just a few days after birth, a newborn will recognize her mother's smell and will use olfactory (smell) cues to locate the mother's nipple. The various foods ingested by the mother during pregnancy result in a liquid diet of different tastes, with the amniotic fluid typically being sweet. No surprise then that a fussy baby is often soothed by sugar water. Infants typically dislike sour tastes and fail to respond to salty tastes until around four months of age.

Some kids are miraculously open to eating everything. But quite often, toddlers become selective about what they will and will not eat. As the taste buds and smell receptors develop and the child experiences new aromas and flavors, and observes family and friends trying "weird" foods, he'll try new things.

Of course, the nose smells much more than food. It is a primitive sense that alerts us to danger; we can smell smoke before we see it, for example. Indeed, everything and everyone smells. Babies mouth just about everything as a means of exploring their new world, including hands, teethers, toys, dishware, furniture, and more. In doing so, they are simultaneously picking up smell information that is carried passively on air currents. Specialized smelling cells called olfactory receptors send scent information directly to the limbic system of the brain, which is the seat of emotion, long-term memory, pleasure, and motivation. Early on the baby tags certain smells (and tastes by association) positively or negatively. By the time they are school aged, kids often have very strong opinions about what smells and tastes great or gross—opinions that may last through adulthood.

As you think about your client's taste and smell processing skills, consider these factors:

- Does your client have a varied food repertoire, including flavors and textures most others enjoy?
- Are there certain foods your client cannot bear to eat or even be around?
- Are there certain foods your client craves?
- Does your client sniff objects in an unusual way?
- What everyday smells does your client find calming versus alarming?
- Are there certain smells your client cannot stand?

So far we've considered the familiar senses that pick up and use input entering your body from the outside world. Several internal senses play extremely important roles in how we feel and function every moment of the day, including the proprioceptive, vestibular, and interoceptive senses. All are quite important to understand when you are helping your clients.

Proprioceptive Sense

If you closed your eyes right now and moved your hand behind your head, or out to the side and around in assorted directions, your brain would know exactly where your hand was positioned without using your vision. Can you accurately bring your fingertips together above your head? Can you tie your shoelaces without looking? Type without looking at your keyboard? Your proprioceptive sense is providing you with internal body awareness, letting you keep track of every part of your body at all times.

Proprioception relies on information derived from sensory receptors in joints, muscles, ligaments, and connective tissue that tell you exactly where your body parts are without you having to see them. As you sit and read this, the joints, muscles, and connective tissue in your legs, hips, and buttocks are compressed. When you get up and move, you elongate certain muscles and contract others, changing the compression forces on joints in your body. If you do some active stretching, you'll lengthen tight muscles and pull the underlying joints apart a bit. If you are thirsty, you might pour yourself some water. As you reach for a glass in the cupboard, your proprioceptive system will work with your visual system to tell your arm muscles how much to stretch, working with your eyes to precisely grade your movements. As you fill your glass, proprioceptors in your arm will detect the increasing weight and alert you to look closely when it's nearly full.

This internal body awareness provides you a mental map of your position in space at all times, kind of like a built-in GPS. It takes time to develop these unsung but miraculous abilities. Movement in the young child is adorably awkward and stiff until he learns to move his body parts smoothly through space. Needless to say, kids can be quite clumsy, spilling milk, breaking crayons, tripping over their own feet, bumping into furniture or other children in preschool. Moving breakables out of reach and cushioning hard edges become reflex actions for most new parents.

The playground is a wonderful place to build proprioceptive skills as kids climb up ladders, jump on chain bridges, hang upside down from monkey bars, and so on. The more they move through space and engage with people, toys, tools, and objects in the environment, the better they become at using just the right amount of force. When learning new motor challenges, they first rely greatly on vision to guide their movements, looking carefully at their fingers when learning to form letters and tie their shoelaces, watching their feet when learning to dance or skate, and becoming disoriented when playing pin the tail on the donkey with a blindfold on. Later they can do these things with increased reliance on proprioception. They learn how to make adjustments to throw a curve ball and to tie hair back in a braid without looking in a mirror. The child who once cried her parents awake to help her get to the bathroom during the night eventually learns to navigate herself there without even turning the lights on, relying on her body awareness coupled with her spatial memory of her bedroom, the hallway, and the bathroom.

As you think about your client's proprioceptive processing skills, consider these factors:

• Does your client seem clumsy or physically awkward?

• Do his movements seem hesitant or stiff?

• Does she enjoy toys that require the use of force, such as pop beads, clay, Legos, or other construction toys?

• Is her handwriting or coloring very light or dark?

• Does he enjoy new physical challenges such as learning to skate or swim?

Vestibular Sense

Whenever you change your head position—nod yes or no, do a pirouette, ski down a hill, ride in a car or airplane—vestibular receptors in your inner ear receive important information about movement and gravitational changes. This enables you to maintain your balance, move efficiently against gravity, maintain appropriate muscle tone, and feel safe and secure physically and emotionally. By telling us which way is up at all times, the vestibular sense helps keep our world and our bodies in equilibrium.

The vestibular system is hard at work 24/7 since the downward pull of gravity is constant. In the womb, babies float around and learn to move in a confined space, stimulating vestibular receptors located in the inner ears. As they develop, most kids love engaging in vestibular play, including going down playground slides, playing on swings, spinning, running, doing somersaults, and hanging upside down from the jungle gym. Our vestibular receptors make working against the force of gravity and moving through space fun and easy.

The vestibular apparatus is quite complex and sophisticated. It consists of otolithic organs and semicircular canals. The otolithic organs—the utricle and saccule—detect linear acceleration (speeding up) and deceleration (slowing down). These organs are lined with tiny hairs called cilia that are embedded in a gelatinous goo containing calcium carbonate crystals called otoconia. In response to acceleration such as a car speeding up, the cilia bend and displace the crystals, providing you with vital sensory information about direction, intensity of gravity, and speed of movement. If you slowly creep forward in your car, your otoliths indicate that you are going forward, that the movement is not fast, and that the gravitational forces are minimal. However, if you are in an airplane taking off, your otoliths alert you that you are going extremely quickly and that intense gravitational forces are at work.

Meanwhile, the semicircular canals in the inner ear detect rotation, a different type of movement. These three fluid-filled canals are at roughly right angles to each other. As you move, the fluid moves too, pushing on a structure called the cupula that contains hair cells that convert the mechanical movement into electrical signals. Rotational movement such as spinning around affects one canal, while up-and-down movement like nodding your head affects another, while side-to-side movements such as doing cartwheels affect the third canal. Working in tandem with the visual and proprioceptive sensory systems, the vestibular system helps us to balance, maintain muscle tone, move against gravity, and keep the world in visual focus as we move.

The vestibulo-ocular reflex keeps an image stable on the retinas of the eyes by keeping it in the center of the visual field. To see how this works, look at the word *focus* and turn your head to the left. You may notice that your eyes move to the right to stay on the word. Visual-vestibular integration helps keep the visual field stable while you move, letting you watch TV while running on a treadmill or letting a child keep eye contact with you as she jumps up and down on a trampoline.

The vestibular system functions like a gyroscope to tell you how your head and body are oriented in space, integrating seamlessly with proprioceptors in your muscles, joints, and connective tissues so you can counteract the force of gravity. Consider riding a bicycle. If you tilt to the right, your left-side muscles kick in to pull you upright. Otherwise, you would simply continue tilting to the right until you fell down. In this way, the vestibular system has a direct, powerful influence on muscle tone and posture by telling muscles how much they need to contract and relax in order to stay upright and move against the constant downward pull of gravity.

The ability to balance and move against gravity are an essential part of development. As a child masters rolling over, walking, running, jumping, riding a bicycle, skating, and more, he learns to work with his vestibular system to stay aligned in space so he feels physically safe and secure on the planet. Proprioceptors and vestibular receptors work together to make it possible for a child to adjust movements when stepping from the sidewalk onto grass, walking in snow, jumping off a diving board, coming to the surface of the water, or swimming to the edge of a pool.

As you think about your client's vestibular processing skills, consider these factors:

- What is the client's movement like? Does he seek out novel movement experiences such as amusement park rides, or avoid them?
- Does she enjoy going to the playground? Does she actively play on climbing equipment, slides, and swings? Or does she prefer the sandbox?
- Does the older child engage in athletic activities? Or does he prefer more sedentary activities like reading and watching TV?
- What are her gym class and recess time like?
- Does he get dizzy easily or rarely? Carsick? Seasick?
- Does she become disoriented when she bends over?
- Does he seem to crave movement? Seem to be always on the go?
- Does she seem kind of lethargic or even lazy?

The Interoceptive Sense

The interoceptive sense is an internal body sense that detects essential regulation responses for body functions including heart rate, respiration, blood pressure, hunger, thirst, temperature, and bowel and bladder sensations.

These body-based feelings, largely experienced at the border of consciousness, complete the picture of how we experience our bodies and define our place in the world. They play an essential role in our state of arousal, feelings, emotions, and self-awareness. When interoceptive messages reach our consciousness, they can have a strong impact. The client who becomes aware of a rapid heartbeat and increased blood pressure will need to judge whether it is proportional to the experience of jogging, for example, or whether she needs to take some kind of action to reduce these visceral responses. If a person becomes aware he is running a fever, he needs to monitor it and take necessary steps to feel better.

Most of the time, most of us are not consciously aware of interoceptive input such as how fast our heart is beating or how fast we are breathing unless something happens to increase these rates. For the person with increased sensitivity to these things, having basic involuntary functions such as heartbeat and respiration within conscious awareness can produce anxiety. Difficulties processing hunger and satiety can result in feeding problems and eating disorders. Children who cannot tell when they have to use the bathroom may have frequent accidents even when they have developed sphincter control because they simply cannot feel the need to go.

As you think about your client's interoceptive processing skills, consider these factors:

- Does the child have regular cycles of hunger and satiety?
- Does he know when he is thirsty?
- Did she potty train roughly on schedule? Does she still have accidents?
- Can he tell if he is getting sick?
- How does she respond to increased heart rate during exercise or other physical activity?
- Does he breathe without conscious thought?
- Does she have psychosomatic complaints (Cameron, 2001)?

LIFE IS MULTISENSORY

While it's important to understand each individual sensory system, remember that just about every daily life experience affects just about every sensory system simultaneously. To illustrate, try this experiment: stand up and feel how your body is balancing. Next close your eyes and see if it feels any different. How much did your vision impact your ability to stay upright? Then stand on one foot with your eyes open and see what that feels like. Then close your eyes. Was it harder to maintain your balance in this challenging position without using your vision to stay upright? Probably, because it's all connected.

Let's say a parent takes a child with sensory problems to the supermarket to do the family shopping. Parents of sensitive kids know this is a danger zone, but often do not understand why. In fact, in such environments, every sensory system is affected:

- Touch: feeling the shopping cart handlebar, touching vegetables and fruit, boxes, cans, handling money, feeling the colder temperature in the dairy aisle, becoming overheated if dressed for cold weather outside, and more.
- Sound: hearing overhead announcements and music, people talking, shopping carts rolling, and more.
- Sight: scanning visually crowded shelves and displays, people moving, reflections of fluorescent lighting on flooring, and more.
- Smell: food, disinfectants, cleaning products, and more.
- Taste: aftertaste in mouth from food and beverages ingested previously, food samples, and possibly more.
- Proprioceptive: pushing the weight of the cart or carrying the basket, pushing and turning while navigating aisles, lifting items of various sizes, and more.
- Vestibular: walking, stopping and starting, bending, and reaching to obtain items and more.
- Interoceptive: monitoring internal body state at all times, largely outside of conscious thought unless some issue needs to be handled such as going to the bathroom.

Most of us can deal with such multisensory stimulation without a hitch, but people with sensory processing challenges may become overstimulated and overwhelmed in such an environment. Much depends on the individual's unique sensory threshold, that is, how sensitive he is to potentially irritating stimuli such as loud noises, bright lights, unfamiliar textures, and strong tastes. Sensory threshold is, of course, is a widely accepted temperamental trait (Thomas, Chess, & Birch, 1968; Turecki, 2000), along with:

- Activity level: The degree of body activity and movement. Is the child always active and physically busy or more sedentary?
- Biological regularity: The degree of regular eating, sleeping, and bowel habits. Are hunger, sleep, and elimination cycles predictable?
- Adaptability: How quickly can the child adapt to changes in routine or overcome an initial negative response?
- Approach/withdrawal: How does the child react to new people or unfamiliar situations? Is the child outgoing or shy?
- Intensity: To what degree does the child react strongly, either positively or negatively, to situations?
- Mood: Does the child have a predominantly positive or negative mood? To what extent is the child pleasant and cheerful or unpleasant and sad?
- Distractibility: How easily is the child distracted? Is the child able to block out external stimuli?
- Persistence/attention span: How long will the child continue with an activity? Does the child give up when there is a problem or keep trying? Does the child maintain focus or does the child's mind wander?

CHAPTER 2

Screening for Sensitivities

All of us have sensory preferences and intolerances. Perhaps you can't bear the feeling of wool against your skin and only wear cotton. Perhaps you cannot tolerate hip-hop music and instead listen to music with slow, steady rhythm and gentle harmonies. Perhaps the idea of going on a roller coaster, bungee jumping, or skydiving repels you. You might prefer a scenic boat ride or going for a hike in the woods. And while you may enjoy spending time with friends, perhaps you would prefer a quiet get-together with a friend or two over a crowded party with loud music. You may not be an adventurous eater and have a strong preference for familiar comfort foods. If you are more of a sensory seeker, on the other hand, you may crave adventure, prefer intense, fast movement and more upbeat music, and thrive on new, stimulating experiences.

As we mature, we learn what kinds of sensory input we like and dislike and make choices about who we are and what we do with our time.

As adults, we are generally able to control our environments in a way that matches our sensory needs. You buy clothing that feels most comfortable. You install dimmer switches if you want to control how bright the lighting is. You may go for a run in the morning if that helps you feel ready to face the day. When work becomes stressful, you might take a break, sip some water, or have a cup of coffee to keep going. Even if you are stuck in a dull meeting, you can excuse yourself to go to the bathroom, chew gum, or doodle surreptitiously.

In contrast, children have little opportunity to adjust the environment to meet their needs. If they are overstimulated by the noise and chaos of drop-off time at school, they can't just show up late every day. If they are bothered by the glare of overhead fluorescents, they can't simply turn the lights off.

Ideally, home and school environments are a good match with the child. After all, most kids learn to adapt fairly easily to new people and new situations. The problem is when the child struggles to process sensory demands. The greater the mismatch between sensory needs and the environment, the greater the challenge and potential discomfort and poor behavioral reactions.

If overwhelmed—or underaroused—by the constant stream of sensory input that comes with being alive, a person may struggle with learning, playing, self-care, socializing, and overall physical and psychological development.

Like so many things, sensory problems run on a continuum. At the milder end, the fussy child who avoids getting messy with glue or paint and will wear only very soft clothing and has a limited repertoire of acceptable foods may naturally grow out of it, especially with some desensitization of the skin and slow, patient introduction of new foods.

A child who gets edgy when classmates are nearby because she is anxious about being touched or pushed, who cannot tolerate the smell or texture of most foods, who becomes overstimulated easily and has frequent meltdowns, needs some help. Toward the middle of the sensory issues continuum, there is increasing difficulty, often in the form of acting out and tuning out behaviors that require more intensive intervention. The diagnosis of sensory processing disorder (SPD) becomes relevant when sensory differences interfere with everyday function. Toward the more severe end of the continuum, sensory problems become increasingly disabling. This is most often seen in people with neurobehavioral disorders such as autism, who may be in a constant state of vigilance, experiencing sights, sounds, and other input as annoying or truly painful, along with sensory overload, sensory jumbling, and actual sensory whiteouts.

Consider these children. Tyler is a preschooler who enjoys all kinds of sensory input: hugs and kisses, rough-and-tumble play, listening to fun music, bouncing and rocking on his Rody horse, trying different foods, and smelling interesting aromas. His parents note his likes and dislikes, try to protect him from unpleasant sensations, and do their best to present him with novelty and excitement while avoiding overstimulation. Tyler has learned early on that the world is a safe place where his parents will come to his aid when he is distressed. As he matures, this sense of security will help him to comfort himself as needed while he explores his world.

Next, let's consider Tyler's younger brother, Max. His parents noticed early on that Max responds differently than Tyler to new experiences. Max becomes agitated when he sees unfamiliar toys, especially those that make noise, as well as new people, especially women who speak in high-pitched, animated voices. He cries when taken to toddler gymnastics and when put in the baby swings at the playground. He gets upset when people laugh or clap and praise him. He gags and sometimes vomits when he smells certain foods such as eggs and bananas. He wakes up crying most nights and can't fall back asleep unless a parent sleeps with him.

Their parents marvel at how different the boys are. Tyler craves playing with his friends at school but Max is happiest playing alone with blocks. Their parents are sad to keep them separated so much of the time, but Max lashes out at friendly advances from his brother, hitting and even biting him if he doesn't back off instantly. His parents recognize that they have to use completely different parenting styles with easygoing, playful Tyler and with hypervigilant, self-contained Max.

Next, let's consider Lily, who is swaddled in her orphanage crib most of the day in a dimly lit room along with six other infants. Lily receives meals through a bottle propped in her mouth and is picked up only for diaper changes a few times a day by a caregiver who says little to her. When Lily is adopted at 8 months old, she is showered with affection by her new parents, encounters bright light and several adults talking animatedly, feels wind and sun on her skin, eats unfamiliar food, and smells flowers, baby powder, and other completely alien things. It's a whole new world for Lily, and she is cautious and bewildered. As her parents get to know her, they learn to recognize when she is becoming stressed, and learn to slow down and follow her lead. As she increasingly attaches to her parents and learns that the sensations she is experiencing are not threatening to her, she becomes more self-assured and ready to check out her interesting new world. Even so, Lily remains slow to warm up to new people and places, is anxious in busy environments like the playground and parties, and has not made any real friends. While everyone agrees she is a bright child, she is scheduled for psychoeducational testing because she just can't keep up academically now that she is in fourth grade.

Finally, let's consider Rosie, an 18-year-old with autism. Rosie has come a long way through hundreds of hours of specialized teaching and therapy over the years, including occupational therapy, physical therapy, and speech-language therapy all supplemented with excellent carryover at home by her loving parents and grandparents. Rosie is now in a transition program to increase her independence with daily life skills such as managing local transportation, interacting with potential future coworkers, and self-advocacy. Even now, she has frequent meltdowns, especially when she is tired. Listening to several people talking at once over a long period, making a lot of transitions from one activity to another, and spending more than a short time in busy, crowded places like the shopping mall can send her into a tailspin. As high functioning as she is, Rosie will still bang her head, pull her hair, and scream when she becomes dysregulated. Rosie's current occupational therapist (OT) and psychologist are helping her to develop greater self-awareness so she can recognize warning signs and act quickly to prevent sensory overload and meltdowns.

WHAT'S GOING ON?

It's essential to consider a wide swath of issues, including innate temperament, current emotional state, physical health, executive function, and, yes, sensory differences, when you are attempting to understand and help a child, teen, or adult.

As you know, sensory differences range from personality quirks that are no big deal to more serious deficits that need to be thoroughly evaluated and addressed. The Sensory Screening Tool in this chapter will help you develop a clearer picture of how kids experience sensory input at home, at school, and in the community.

One of the marvelous things about screening tools is that they initiate important conversations. All too often, parents bring their concerns to the pediatrician who tells them not to worry or to simply wait and see. This is usually not helpful or at all reassuring to parents who know on a gut level that something is just not right with their child.

Pediatricians typically see patients for a short examination in the office where the child may be intimidated and frightened. This does not represent a true picture of what is going on in daily life. While most pediatricians ask parents about sleep, eating, and bowel habits, they usually do not ask open-ended questions about daily quality-of-life issues such as what it's like to get ready for school in the morning, do homework, or go to the playground.

As a clinician, you may well be the first person who asks questions about the quality of the child's daily life in sensory terms. You may be the first person to ask parents about what happens when the child gets a haircut, for example. A parent might report to the pediatrician that the child detests getting his hair cut. Not a big deal to the pediatrician, who knows many kids hate haircuts. But you may well find out that the child requires both parents to pin him down, a video to watch, and the promise of an ice cream sundae afterward.

USING THE SENSORY SCREENING TOOL

The home-based section of the Sensory Screening Tool should be filled out by parents or caregivers who know the child well. It is ideal for parents to fill it out together. Encourage them to note any discrepancies between their answers as this can yield valuable clues. For example, a child may be more cooperative getting dressed with one parent present rather than the other. Maybe that parent does something special such as giving a brisk morning massage or laying out clothing the night before. If there is a babysitter who spends a lot of time with the child, you can ask her to fill out a copy as well. If the child lives in a group home, ask the person who is most involved in the child's care to complete the screening.

The school-based section should be filled out by the classroom teacher as well as the special education itinerant teacher (SEIT) or paraprofessional if the student has one. As you'll read in Chapter 5, a SEIT is a specialized instructor that may work with a student with special learning and/or behavioral needs. Again, it's ideal for the teaching team to fill out the Sensory Screening Tool together, noting any discrepancies, or you can give each person a copy.

Please feel free to duplicate the Sensory Screening Tool in this book or you can download it from sensoryprocessingchallenges.com.

SENSORY SCREENING TOOL: HOME

Child's Name: _____

Your Name: _____

Relationship to Child: _____

Child's Age: _____

Date: _____

Touch Sense	Always	Sometimes	Rarely	Never	Unsure/Not Applicable
Objects to washing face, hair, or body	O	O	O	O	O
Reacts negatively to unexpected touch	O	O	O	O	O
Dislikes light touch	O	O	O	O	O
Dislikes brushing teeth	O	O	O	O	O
Objects to getting haircuts	O	O	O	O	O
Resists nail trimming	O	O	O	O	O
Dislikes certain clothing fabrics	O	O	O	O	O
Avoids getting hands or face messy	O	O	O	O	O
Dislikes or insists on wearing socks	O	O	O	O	O
Insists on or refuses to wear shoes, sneakers, sandals, or boots	O	O	O	O	O
Avoids or excessively craves physical contact such as hugs, cuddles, and kisses	O	O	O	O	O
Frequently touches or fidgets with toys or other objects	O	O	O	O	O
Craves or avoids certain food textures, such as dry, slippery, chewy, crunchy, or mixed	O	O	O	O	O
Mouths nonfood objects such as hands, clothing, toys	O	O	O	O	O

	Always	Sometimes	Rarely	Never	Unsure/Not Applicable
Particular about pajamas and bed linens	O	O	O	O	O
Unusually aware or unaware of changes in temperature	O	O	O	O	O
Seem oversensitive or undersensitive to minor injuries	O	O	O	O	O
Engages in repetitive tactile behaviors such as tapping, rubbing, squeezing, banging	O	O	O	O	O

Additional notes and observations:

Sound Sense

	Always	Sometimes	Rarely	Never	Unsure/Not Applicable
Unusually distressed by sounds such as alarms, thunder, blender, vacuum, hair dryer, toilet flush	O	O	O	O	O
Dislikes noisy settings such as a busy playground, party, restaurant, or store	O	O	O	O	O
Watches TV or listens to music at very high or very low volume	O	O	O	O	O
Makes unusual sounds	O	O	O	O	O
Doesn't consistently respond to someone speaking to him	O	O	O	O	O
Unable to concentrate in noisy places	O	O	O	O	O
Difficulty sleeping if there is any noise	O	O	O	O	O
Has delays in expressive or receptive language	O	O	O	O	O
Speaks very loudly or quietly	O	O	O	O	O
Avoids live or recorded music	O	O	O	O	O

	Always	Sometimes	Rarely	Never	Unsure/Not Applicable
Seems to mishear what is being said; for example, confuses words or ideas	○	○	○	○	○
Engages in repetitive auditory behaviors such as humming, repeating, and making noises	○	○	○	○	○

Additional notes and observations:

Vision Sense

	Always	Sometimes	Rarely	Never	Unsure/Not Applicable
Squints, blinks, or rubs eyes frequently	○	○	○	○	○
Makes poor eye contact	○	○	○	○	○
Uses peripheral vision to look at things	○	○	○	○	○
Has trouble finding items in busy visual fields such as a toy in toy chest or coat in a closet	○	○	○	○	○
Struggles with reading	○	○	○	○	○
Take excessive time to complete written work	○	○	○	○	○
Distressed by sunlight, glare, bright light, fluorescent lighting	○	○	○	○	○
Craves or avoids very colorful, active computer and video games and TV shows	○	○	○	○	○
Distressed by or prefers dim lighting or being in the dark	○	○	○	○	○
Struggles to follow objects or people as they move	○	○	○	○	○
Has difficulty with ball skills such as catching and throwing	○	○	○	○	○
Gets overwhelmed easily in crowded environments such as the playground and stores	○	○	○	○	○

	Always	Sometimes	Rarely	Never	Unsure/Not Applicable
Engages in repetitive visual behaviors such as blinking, spinning objects, flapping hands, flicking fingers in front of eyes, turning lights on and off	O	O	O	O	O

Additional notes and observations:

Taste and Smell Sense

	Always	Sometimes	Rarely	Never	Unsure/Not Applicable
Avoids or complains about certain smells	O	O	O	O	O
Smells nonfood items such as people and objects	O	O	O	O	O
Avoids foods most children enjoy	O	O	O	O	O
Seeks out or avoids strongly flavored foods (spicy, salty, sweet, or sour)	O	O	O	O	O
Has a limited food repertoire	O	O	O	O	O
Resists trying new foods	O	O	O	O	O
Gags or gets nauseated when presented with certain foods or smells	O	O	O	O	O
Acts out at mealtime	O	O	O	O	O
Mouths or licks objects and people	O	O	O	O	O

Additional notes and observations:

Movement and Body Senses

	Always	Sometimes	Rarely	Never	Unsure/Not Applicable
Seems restless or always on the move	O	O	O	O	O
Seems lethargic or hard to engage	O	O	O	O	O

	Always	Sometimes	Rarely	Never	Unsure/Not Applicable
Avoids changes in head position	O	O	O	O	O
Seems clumsy—walks or runs awkwardly, drops or breaks things frequently	O	O	O	O	O
Unusually cautious when climbing stairs	O	O	O	O	O
Fidgets with objects and clothing	O	O	O	O	O
Touches furniture or walls when walking	O	O	O	O	O
Gets dizzy easily or never seems to get dizzy	O	O	O	O	O
Avoids or craves using playground equipment such as slides and swings	O	O	O	O	O
Doesn't seem to know where body parts are—bumps into toys, furniture, walls	O	O	O	O	O
Uses too much or too little force on pencils, crayons, or markers; for example, marks are very heavy or light, breaks crayons	O	O	O	O	O
Accidentally spills when opening containers, pouring, or drinking	O	O	O	O	O
Crashes and falls seemingly on purpose	O	O	O	O	O
Engages in repetitive movements such as rocking, jumping, spinning	O	O	O	O	O

Additional notes and observations:

Behavior, Emotions, Play, and Self-Care

	Always	Sometimes	Rarely	Never	Unsure/Not Applicable
Craves predictability and familiarity	O	O	O	O	O
Stops working to look at what others are doing	O	O	O	O	O
Struggles with sequencing activities	O	O	O	O	O

	Always	Sometimes	Rarely	Never	Unsure/Not Applicable
Poor organization, loses things frequently	○	○	○	○	○
Has difficulty with transitions such as from playing to going outdoors or getting ready for school	○	○	○	○	○
Engages in repetitive play	○	○	○	○	○
Doesn't seem to understand concept of personal space	○	○	○	○	○
Has difficulty playing with siblings or other children	○	○	○	○	○
Easily overwhelmed or frustrated	○	○	○	○	○
Frequently tunes out or withdraws	○	○	○	○	○
Frequently acts out or has tantrums	○	○	○	○	○
Needs reminders to follow household or school rules and routines	○	○	○	○	○
Has difficulty making friends	○	○	○	○	○
Cries more easily than others of same age	○	○	○	○	○
Has difficulty falling asleep, staying asleep, and/or waking up	○	○	○	○	○
Unpredictable hunger cycles	○	○	○	○	○
Seems less independent than children of same age	○	○	○	○	○

Additional notes and observations:

Please return your completed Sensory Screening Tool to:

SENSORY SCREENING TOOL: SCHOOL

Student's Name: _____

Grade: _____

Your Name: _____

Your Title: _____

Date: _____

Touch Sense	Always	Sometimes	Rarely	Never	Unsure/Not Applicable
Avoids casual touch from classmates or teachers	O	O	O	O	O
Becomes "silly" (giggly or babyish) or annoyed when touched	O	O	O	O	O
Seeks excessive physical contact with others	O	O	O	O	O
Avoids or seeks out messy materials such as glue, clay, paint, and sand	O	O	O	O	O
Insists on cleaning hands immediately when messy	O	O	O	O	O
Distracted by clothing or shoes	O	O	O	O	O
Chews or sucks on clothing, hands, pencils, or other objects	O	O	O	O	O
Craves or avoids hot or cold items	O	O	O	O	O
Dislikes or craves certain textures—fabric, paper, toys, and so on	O	O	O	O	O
Disturbed by vibration, such as from air conditioner or truck	O	O	O	O	O
Dislikes being physically close to classmates; for example, avoids standing in line	O	O	O	O	O
Seems oversensitive or undersensitive to minor injuries	O	O	O	O	O

	Always	Sometimes	Rarely	Never	Unsure/Not Applicable
Engages in repetitive tactile behaviors such as tapping, rubbing, squeezing, banging	O	O	O	O	O

Additional notes and observations:

Sound Sense

	Always	Sometimes	Rarely	Never	Unsure/Not Applicable
Distressed by loud noises such as fire drill, gym whistle, PA announcements	O	O	O	O	O
Disturbed by sounds such as singing and musical instruments	O	O	O	O	O
Complains that other people, music, or other sounds are too loud	O	O	O	O	O
Speaks with an unusually loud or quiet voice	O	O	O	O	O
Doesn't seem to hear you or ignores you	O	O	O	O	O
Seems to mishear what is being said, for example, confuses words or ideas	O	O	O	O	O
Can't focus when there is noise in the room	O	O	O	O	O
Frequent outbursts or withdrawal in gym, recess, cafeteria, or assemblies	O	O	O	O	O
Learns more easily one-on-one than in a group	O	O	O	O	O
Engages in repetitive auditory behaviors such as humming, repeating, and making noises	O	O	O	O	O

Additional notes and observations:

Vision Sense

	Always	Sometimes	Rarely	Never	Unsure/Not Applicable
Squints, blinks, or rubs eyes frequently	○	○	○	○	○
Makes poor eye contact	○	○	○	○	○
Uses peripheral vision to look at things	○	○	○	○	○
Struggles with reading	○	○	○	○	○
Has difficulty with eye-hand coordination activities	○	○	○	○	○
Difficulty copying from the board	○	○	○	○	○
Has trouble completing age-appropriate jigsaw puzzles	○	○	○	○	○
Annoyed by sunlight, glare, bright light, fluorescent lighting	○	○	○	○	○
Distressed by dim lights or being in the dark	○	○	○	○	○
Struggles to follow objects or people as they move	○	○	○	○	○
Has difficulty with ball skills such as catching and throwing	○	○	○	○	○
Gets overwhelmed easily in crowds, such as playgrounds and assemblies	○	○	○	○	○
Engages in repetitive visual behaviors such as blinking, spinning objects, flapping hands, or flicking fingers in front of eyes	○	○	○	○	○

Additional notes and observations:

Smell and Taste

	Always	Sometimes	Rarely	Never	Unsure/Not Applicable
Seeks out or complains about particular smells	O	O	O	O	O
Smells nonfood items such as people and objects	O	O	O	O	O
Avoids foods most classmates enjoy	O	O	O	O	O
Has a limited food repertoire	O	O	O	O	O
Mouths or licks objects and people	O	O	O	O	O
Gags or gets nauseated when presented with certain foods or smells	O	O	O	O	O
Acts out at snack time or in cafeteria	O	O	O	O	O

Additional notes and observations:

Movement and Body Senses

	Always	Sometimes	Rarely	Never	Unsure/Not Applicable
Seems restless or always on the move	O	O	O	O	O
Seems lethargic or hard to engage	O	O	O	O	O
Avoids changes in head position	O	O	O	O	O
Seems clumsy, walks or runs awkwardly	O	O	O	O	O
Unusually cautious when climbing stairs	O	O	O	O	O
Fidgets with objects and clothing	O	O	O	O	O

	Always	Sometimes	Rarely	Never	Unsure/Not Applicable
Touches furniture or walls when walking	O	O	O	O	O
Gets dizzy easily or never seems to get dizzy	O	O	O	O	O
Avoids or craves using playground equipment such as slides and swings	O	O	O	O	O
Doesn't seem to know where body parts are—bumps into toys, furniture, walls, or other students	O	O	O	O	O
Uses too much or too little force on pencils, crayons, or markers; for example, marks are very heavy or light, breaks crayons	O	O	O	O	O
Accidentally spills when opening containers, pouring, or drinking	O	O	O	O	O
Struggles to remain seated	O	O	O	O	O
Crashes and falls seemingly on purpose	O	O	O	O	O
Engages in repetitive movement such as spinning, rocking, jumping	O	O	O	O	O

Additional notes and observations:

Behavior, Learning, and Social Issues

	Always	Sometimes	Rarely	Never	Unsure/Not Applicable
Difficulty initiating and completing tasks	O	O	O	O	O
Stops working to look at what others are doing	O	O	O	O	O
Struggles with sequencing activities	O	O	O	O	O
Poor organization, loses things frequently	O	O	O	O	O
Craves predictability	O	O	O	O	O

	Always	Sometimes	Rarely	Never	Unsure/Not Applicable
Has difficulty with transitions between activities	○	○	○	○	○
Engages in repetitive play	○	○	○	○	○
Doesn't seem to understand concept of personal space	○	○	○	○	○
Has difficulty joining group activities	○	○	○	○	○
Easily overwhelmed or frustrated	○	○	○	○	○
Frequently tunes out or withdraws	○	○	○	○	○
Frequently acts out or has tantrums	○	○	○	○	○
Cries more easily than classmates	○	○	○	○	○
Needs frequent reminders to follow class rules and routines	○	○	○	○	○
Has difficulty making friends	○	○	○	○	○
Struggles with handwriting	○	○	○	○	○
Struggles with fine motor skills such as using scissors and clothing fasteners	○	○	○	○	○
Seems to have low self-esteem	○	○	○	○	○

Additional notes and observations:

Please return your completed Sensory Screening Tool to:

MAKING SENSE OF THE RESULTS

As you review the results of the Sensory Screening Tool, you will develop a picture of how the child functions at home and at school from a sensory standpoint. You may need to get clarification during a follow-up meeting with the parents and teachers. Ideally, you will also have a chance to observe the child in natural settings such as at home, at school, and on the playground.

Most children have a few mild sensitivities, denoted on the Sensory Screening Tool by Rarely or even a few Sometimes. As you review the completed screening, note the frequency of Always and Sometimes. Also note which sensory systems have greater numbers of Always and Sometimes.

Responses that tend toward Sometimes and Always indicate increasingly significant sensory differences. Part II of this book provides an overview of interventions and treatment strategies that therapists who work with kids should be familiar with, but if a child's ratings on the Sensory Screening Tool fall primarily in the Sometimes and Always categories, it's best to refer the child to a specialist. You'll read about collaborating with occupational therapists (OTs) in Chapter 5.

As a general guideline for your response to the results of the tool, you need have no special concern about a child who has from zero to two ratings of Always or Sometimes in each section. You can certainly recommend strategies for any noted sensory difficulties, for example, seamless socks if the child refuses to wear socks. You'll find such interventions throughout this book, especially in Chapters 6 and 7.

A child who has three or more ratings of Always or Sometimes in one or more sections should be referred for evaluation by an OT with advanced training and experience in sensory processing challenges. The evaluating OT will assess the child's sensory processing skills along with neuromuscular development, fine and gross motor skills, motor planning (praxis) skills, visual perceptual, self-help skills, and visual-motor integration abilities. You can begin helping the client to develop insight into the challenges and recommend sensory strategies that may be of immediate help.

CHAPTER 3

What Is Sensory Processing Disorder?

Efficient sensory processing creates the foundation for a sense of physical safety and emotional security and empowers us to confidently explore how our bodies interact with the world. Sensory processing is something most of us do automatically, without conscious effort, and most of us do it quite proficiently.

Unfortunately, this process does not always work well. Some people have differences in how their sensory receptors receive input, how their nerves send sensory information to the brain, and how their brain perceives it, decides whether or not to react, and then guides the response.

A young child may refuse to use the playground swing because she fell off once and is hesitant to try it again. She may be comfortable if her parent holds her while she is swinging fairly low to the ground, starting and stopping whenever she requests it so she regains a sense of control and mastery. A child with sensory issues may refuse to use the playground swing because it feels like she is bungee jumping into outer space, with the whole world moving along with her.

Variations in sensory processing skills can have a huge impact on how kids experience and interact with the world. When sensory processing differences interfere with everyday function, a diagnosis of sensory processing disorder (SPD) should be considered.

HOW DOES SPD PLAY OUT IN REAL LIFE?

When I am overstimulated, it feels like there is an energy surge in my body and ants are crawling all over me. I feel like I need to get out of my skin. Imagine not feeling safe in your own body—the one place you should always feel safe in! Feeling safe is not always the case for individuals with sensory processing challenges and autism like me. (Chloe Rothschild, 21-year-old autism advocate)

Some days everything hurts me. It seems like everyone is yelling in my ears and my body feels on edge and I can't stay still. It feels like my eyes are burning with chemicals. I just want to get home, take my clothes off, and get into my bed under a heavy blanket in the dark. I cry a lot and then after a little while I feel like I can be a part of the world again. (tenth grader)

There's this constant low-grade buzzing in my ears and my bones. If I run around, jump on a trampoline, or do some really intense exercise, that makes me feel good for a while. (second grader)

My clothes hurt me. (kindergartner)

While SPD is a term that has only recently become familiar to some clinicians, parents, teachers, pediatricians, and others, sensory processing impairments have long been recognized as a symptom of stroke, multiple sclerosis, and other medical conditions. Dr. A. Jean Ayres, an OT, recognized and explored how sensory processing deficits interfered with development and learning in her clinical pediatric work and pioneered sensory integrative theory and practice for this population. Lorna Jean King (1974), another OT, had great success in applying sensory integrative principles to adults with chronic schizophrenia as well as children with autism to help them improve the nervous system's ability to process sensory input in a more typical way.

Occupational therapists, neurologists, psychologists, and others have continued to build on sensory integration theory and practice. In 2007, Dr. Lucy Jane Miller and her colleagues introduced new terminology for greater diagnostic clarity, which incorporates the same terms used by professionals in other fields (Miller, Anzalone, Lane,

Cermak, & Osten, 2007). The term sensory processing disorder is now widely accepted and used along with sensory integration disorder.

The jury is still out on just how many people are affected by sensory processing problems. A study based on parent perceptions suggested that 5–13 percent of preschool children are affected by SPD in their daily life (Ahn, Miller, Milberger, & McIntosh, 2004). The rates are dramatically higher among people diagnosed with autism, fragile X, ADHD, mood disorders, and other comorbid conditions, which are discussed later in this chapter. A longitudinal study by members of the Sensory Processing Disorder Scientific Work Group, composed of developmental psychologists, clinical psychologists, OTs, pediatric neurologists, and others, found that 16.5 percent of school-age children experience clinically significant sensory overresponsiveness to tactile and auditory stimuli affecting everyday social-emotional function (Ben-Sasson, Carter, & Briggs-Gowan, 2009). More research clearly lies ahead to determine prevalence across diagnoses as well as throughout the life span (see "Risk Factors for SPD" and "Comorbid Conditions" later in this chapter.

SPD BASICS

SPD is an umbrella term that covers three major classifications: sensory modulation disorder, sensory-based motor disorder, and sensory discrimination disorder. A child, teen, or adult may have one or any combination of these sensory processing challenges. For example, a child may have only a sensory modulation problem such as oversensitivity to sounds or visual stimuli or may also have difficulty with postural control as well as discriminating between sensory input experiences.

Sensory Modulation Disorder

Sensory modulation refers to the process by which the central nervous system adjusts neural messages about the intensity, frequency, duration, complexity, and novelty of sensory stimuli. This complex process enables the person to engage in adaptive behavior, ideally responding in proportion to the sensory experience. A person with sensory modulation problems has responses that are out of proportion, responding disproportionately, adversely, or not at all.

Let's say you are driving and hear a fire truck blaring its siren somewhere behind you. The well-modulated response would be to become alert but remain calm, attempt to locate its position, move out of the way, and then drive on once it passes.

Hearing the siren, an overreactive person might respond by becoming nervous with increased breath and heart rate, impulsively jerking the car out of the way, and staying on edge long after the fire truck has passed. An underreactive person may not register that an emergency vehicle is trying to get through traffic until it's right behind him blaring its siren and flashing lights, and only then attempt to get out of the way. Or he may fail to respond entirely and force the fire truck to go around him. Finally, a sensory seeker may be thrilled by this opportunity to zoom through traffic, tailgating the fire truck.

Quite often, it's the child with sensory modulation difficulties—particularly those who are overreactive, for whom everything is too noisy, too uncomfortable, too bright—who is most easily recognized as having sensory processing issues.

Hyper-, Hypo-, and Mixed Reactivity

If a child's skin is so sensitive that certain fabrics and materials hurt, it's no wonder that child will struggle to get dressed and out the door or get changed into pajamas and into bed. If entering a supermarket feels like walking into a rock-and-roll concert with fluorescents flickering on and off like strobe lights, the shopping carts, people, and piped-in music pounding like heavy metal percussion, plus the visual chaos of the food and crowds, it's no wonder a person would become cranky, anxious, or upset. If a child's body is sluggish and floppy like Eeyore's and he uses movement to help wake himself up but then becomes overaroused and disorganized because his nervous system modulates so poorly, it's no wonder he winds up bouncing off the walls like a hyperactive little Tigger.

When sensory processing doesn't work well, nothing works well.

It may help to think of the nervous system as being like an orchestra performing a symphony. All the different instruments—the strings, woodwinds, brass, and percussion—need to be individually in tune, and then must play the right notes at the right volume at the right time in coordination with each other under the conductor's regulating guidance. If an instrument is not properly tuned, plays too loudly or quietly, or out of tempo, or plays a wrong note, the symphony won't sound right. Everyone needs to be in tune, playing the right notes at the right volume at the right time. The conductor uses sensory feedback loops—primarily sound, vibration, and vision—to keep the music beautiful. A person's sensory system is much like an orchestra. When sensory input comes in too loudly or too quietly or gets out of sync, arousal levels, emotions, and behavior get out of whack.

Hypersensitivity (Overreactivity)

If a person is hypersensitive to one or more types of sensory stimulation, his nervous system threshold for sensory input is very low; he requires less intense and less frequent sensory stimuli in order to become aroused enough to respond. It's as if the volume controls are turned up too high on any combination of sensory channels. Global sensory hypersensitivity is often referred to as sensory defensiveness. The hypersensitive person may engage in fight-or-flight behaviors in order to avoid or respond to intolerable sensations. This may take the form of sensory avoidance of those stimuli and lead to withdrawal, limiting participation in social, athletic, and academic activities. It may also take the form of acting out against others who impose on his personal space.

The person with sensory hypersensitivity may become uncomfortable or completely overwhelmed. The same holds true for the person struggling to process multiple sources of input simultaneously, especially over a sustained period of time. The person may resort to monochannel processing, which, in effect, turns off one stream of sensory input while he tunes in to another or, more often, experiences sensory overload, in which he is no longer able to process the input and either tunes out or acts out. You'll read more about this later.

Hyposensitivity (Underreactivity)

If a person is hyposensitive to one or more types of sensory stimulation, her nervous system threshold for sensory input is high; she requires more intense and more frequent sensory stimuli to become aroused enough to respond. It's as if the volume controls aren't turned up enough on any combination of sensory channels. The hypersensitive person may appear sluggish, sleepy, or even lethargic. It may be hard to get this person interested and engaged in an activity or to sustain attention. Some kids may rev themselves up when their nervous system is on such a low idle, and may wind up overexcited and overstimulated.

Mixed Reactivity

Many people with sensory issues have mixed reactivity, reacting strongly to some kinds of input and not much to others. A child with tactile issues may hate wearing certain fabrics but love getting messy with glue and paint. A child may love loud, recorded music yet despise live music at any volume. He may enjoy eating strawberry yogurt one day yet gag at the sight of it on another day.

In fact, one of the hallmarks of SPD is inconsistency, because the nervous system is functioning so inefficiently. For many kids, it depends on whether the input is experienced actively or passively. For example, a child may hate to be hugged but love to give hugs. A child may scream when someone turns on the vacuum cleaner, but be willing to turn it on himself.

Most of us have both good days and bad days. That's typical for everyone. But it tends to be even more touch-and-go for kids with sensory challenges who might have a good morning and a bad afternoon or a good moment and a bad moment depending on what the sensory input is like and how well they are able to handle the experience at that particular moment.

As you think about the kinds of sensory issues your client may be experiencing, keep in mind that sensory problems are highly variable and can change from day to day and context to context. When a person is relaxed, well-fed, and well-rested, bright lights or crowds might not distress him. But when he is under stress due to allergies, a poor diet, and fatigue, walking into a busy store, classroom, or restaurant may throw him into a tailspin.

Sensory-Based Motor Disorder

The person with sensory-based motor issues has difficulty using sensory feedback loops to guide and control movements and posture in order to meet the physical requirements of a motor task. A person with such difficulties may have decreased balance, low muscle tone, and poor strength and endurance as well as motor planning difficulties.

Motor planning refers to the multistep process of deciding what to do, figuring out how to do it, and sequencing the steps to actually execute it. For example, a child on the playground first has to select a piece of equipment to use, such as the monkey bars. Then she needs to figure out how to get up there as well as how to recruit the right body parts to hold on, alternate hands, and swing from bar to bar.

Dyspraxia makes it hard for a child to come up with effective motor plans for unfamiliar tasks and activities. A dyspraxic person struggles with learning new motor planning skills, including gross motor tasks like learning to walk, run, and ride a bicycle, as well as fine motor tasks like buttoning clothing, using scissors, and stringing beads. The dyspraxic child may be awkward, clumsy, and prone to injuries. Dyspraxia can also affect the oral motor planning skills needed to manage the muscles of the mouth for eating and speaking.

Sensory Discrimination Disorder

The person with poor sensory discrimination skills has trouble perceiving the salient features of sensory experiences and may struggle to differentiate between two sources of sensory input. For example, a child may not be able to tell the difference between a pencil and a marker at the bottom of his book bag by touch alone, and may need to see it in order to identify it. The child may not be able to locate where he is being touched and how hard. He may be able to put his T-shirt on but may not pull it all the way down because he cannot sense that it is twisted up around his chest. A child leaning against classmates at circle time may not be aware he is doing this and when pushed away may get upset because he perceives their actions as unwarranted and aggressive.

Many kids with sensory issues take a very long time to get used to something new. When you put on your socks in the morning, you may not even consciously register the sensation. A person with poor habituation would experience those socks as a new sensation for minutes or even hours. Add in the barrage of sensations streaming into the brain all day long and you can imagine how overarousing and overstimulating that would be.

ADDITIONAL SENSORY CHALLENGES

Sensory Processing Disorder and its subtypes are useful classifications. At the same time, sensory issues manifest in different ways for various individuals.

Self-Regulatory Problems

An optimal level of arousal enables a person to participate in activities in an appropriate manner. We are most adaptable and best able to learn when we are in a calm, alert state in which we're not too wired and not too tired. For example, the child who is in an ideal calm, alert state will be able to sit quietly at circle time, listen well, and behave as expected.

Self-regulation refers to the ability to achieve, sustain, and adjust arousal level to meet the demands of activities and situations as they change. The child who self-regulates well can transition easily from a calm, alert state in the classroom to a more physically active, aroused state for playground time, back to calm and alert for dinner and homework, and then to the low-arousal state necessary to drift off to sleep.

It can be hard for kids with sensory issues to tap into that optimal state of arousal. A child with a regulatory disorder has difficulty regulating behavior and physiological, sensory, attentional, motor, or affective processes (DeGangi, 2000). This is often most evident in infancy and early childhood and is correlated with difficult temperament. Note that not every child with SPD has a regulatory disorder. Symptoms of regulatory disorders include poor self-calming with high irritability, sleep and feeding problems, inattention, and mood regulation problems as well as extreme reactions to sensory input. Quite often the child with SPD will have these problems as well. However, not all children with sensory processing challenges have difficulty with issues such as irritability, sleep, feeding, attention, and mood regulation.

Synesthesia

Some people have a condition called synesthesia, in which one sensation conjures up another due to crossover between sensory pathways in the brain. Numbers, letters, or sounds may seem to have colors and tastes may seem to have shapes (Cytowic, 1993). This is a generally benign condition affecting a range of people, including celebrities in the arts and sciences such as Nobel Prize–winning physicist Richard Feynman, writer Vladimir Nabokov, and composer and pianist Duke Ellington.

Monochannel Processing

In contrast, some people have trouble processing input from just one or two sensory channels. They may be supersensitive to noise or easily annoyed by certain textures. They may learn to compensate for these sensitivities and to work around them. Individuals with more significant sensory processing problems become monochannel processors. Just as you would turn down your radio if you were driving and suddenly encountered a traffic jam, a person may need to turn down one source of sensory input in order to tune in to another. For example, a student might avoid looking at the teacher when she is speaking in order to better attend to what she is saying, turning off vision in order to turn on hearing. Or he may be better able to tolerate the oral tactile, taste, and smell sensations that occur while eating if he is in a small quiet room instead of the school cafeteria.

Sensory Overload

Dealing with everyday life experiences that seem unremarkable to most of us can easily overwhelm kids with sensory issues. They may be able to deal with processing demands for a short period or longer if demands are less intense, but if too much demand piles up for too long, the child is at increasing risk of sensory overload.

It may help to think of sensory overload as putting too much food on a flimsy paper plate. Your plate may hold up as you load on a hot dog, potato chips, and some coleslaw, but add potato salad and the whole thing falls apart. You would need to put on less food, get a stronger plate, or both. Similarly, you can use sensory strategies to keep your client feeling comfortable and safe (i.e., reducing sensory load) and reinforce his ability to tolerate greater amounts of sensory challenge.

Consider Rosie. Rosie feels great Saturday morning. Her mom makes cinnamon toast, which is her favorite. She gets to play with her toy ponies and colors a picture too, doing a good job staying inside the lines. Mom does some vacuuming, but that's okay because now Rosie is a big girl and doesn't get upset by the noise any more. She finds the leggings that are comfy, but her Cookie Monster T-shirt is in the wash. She feels sad because that's her lucky shirt.

When Mom fills up the car with gas, Rosie pulls her shirt over her nose and smells her own skin instead. That works pretty well. Then they go downtown for errands, first stopping at the coffee shop for Mom's cappuccino. The coffee smell burns her nose.

Then they go to the big box store to shop. Mom says, "It's still early so it won't be crowded." But the parking lot is crowded, and Rosie still has to get through those sliding glass doors without them shutting and squishing her into spaghetti. She helps Mom find what's on the list, but is worried about getting separated. There are so many people! The overhead announcements are too loud. And the lights are too bright. There is so much stuff to look at. She wants to leave but Mom says they just have to get a few things and check out.

There are hundreds of shoppers and just three registers open and one of the cashiers just walked off for a price check while another is replacing her register paper. That's not fair! The announcements are screaming and Mom stinks like nasty coffee when she says, "Rosie, stay calm and breathe." Rosie can't stay calm. She starts to cry and tries to pull Mom toward the door. Mom says, "Rosie, you need to wait. I'm sorry it's taking so long. After this we'll go to the library where you can look at your animal books." But looking at her daughter, she sees she's gone over the edge. Rosie is a heap on the floor and she's begun to bang her head. Other shoppers are giving Mom dirty looks and one hisses to another, "What a spoiled brat." Mom pays and they get to the car. Both mother and daughter break down in tears.

Life is a multisensory experience that demands that we process multiple sources of sensory input simultaneously. This may be fairly easy if a child is relaxed, well-nourished, and well-rested. However, the intensity and duration of processing involved may require too much energy and effort to sustain. Remember that intensity and duration are relative. Rosie's mom felt that the store was not very crowded or sensory aversive whereas Rosie could not deal with the sensory load or the length of the trip.

Tuning-Out Behaviors

A child may withdraw his attention or engagement from a situation that becomes too much to handle. He may zone out into a self-absorbed state or, as some people have reported, experience sensory static like an old-fashioned TV or even full-blown sensory whiteouts. Hyperfocused behaviors such as lining up toys may help to shut out the unpredictable and perhaps painful outside world and instead to focus on something simple and predictable that he can control.

Acting-Out Behaviors

Rather than avoiding intolerable sensory input, children may respond in ways that are loud or aggressive. They may shout or yell in panic, pain, or anger. They may have a full-blown kicking and screaming tantrum when pushed past their limits. They may throw toys and other objects. They may lash out against others—hitting, kicking, or biting people who are trying to help them or simply in their space. Or such a child may direct acting-out behavior at herself with self-injurious behaviors such as banging her head, biting her hand, picking her scalp, and pulling her hair out.

Stimming Behaviors

Some kids—especially those on the autistic spectrum or with cognitive disabilities—engage in self-stimulatory behaviors such as rocking, spinning, and hand flapping in response to overwhelming sensory processing demands.

It's important to recognize that stimming behaviors run on a continuum. In fact, all of us engage in self-stimulatory behaviors from time to time as a self-soothing mechanism. You may chew gum or drink coffee when you need help staying alert and focused, pump your leg when trying to stay engaged, twirl your hair, rub your ear, or engage in whatever helps you feel and function at your best. We know to keep these stims in check, useful enough to help us, yet subtle enough to be socially acceptable.

The child with significant sensory issues may engage in maladaptive stimming behaviors that can be quite distressing to others in order to:

- Rev up a sluggish nervous system when bored, tired, or understimulated.
- Self-soothe an overwhelmed nervous system.
- Block out overwhelming input.
- Feel better because both self-injurious behaviors and stims release dopamine and endogenous opioids.

For more on repetitive and self-stimulatory behaviors, see Chapter 4.

WHAT THE RESEARCH SHOWS

Sensory processing issues can be upsetting and downright painful for the people who experience them as well as confusing and frustrating for those trying to help. All too often a parent or teacher will view sensory-driven behaviors as something the child would be able to control if only she tried harder, attributing many problems to laziness, stubbornness, being spoiled, being depressed, being high-strung, or having cognitive impairments.

An increasing body of evidence shows that children with SPD have biological differences that make multisensory processing and, therefore, everyday behavioral and emotional responses much more difficult than many realize, including differences in white matter structure, sympathetic and parasympathetic nervous system responses, and poor habituation to sensory stimuli (McIntosh, Miller, Shya, & Hagerman, 1999).

A small but groundbreaking study used diffusion tensor imaging, an advanced form of MRI, to measure the movement of water molecules in the brains of male subjects between the ages of 8 and 11 in order to examine the direction and integrity of white matter fibers which help us to perceive, learn, and think (Owen, Marco, Desai, Fourie, Harris, Hill, Arnett, & Mukherjee, 2013). The study compared 24 typically developing boys with 16 boys diagnosed with SPD but without a diagnosis of autism or prematurity, matching them for gender, age, IQ, and hand dominance. The study found abnormal microstructure of white matter tracts in boys with SPD, primarily in the back of the brain. These posterior cerebral tracts function as neural connectors for auditory, visual, and tactile information and are essential to sensory processing. The study found decreased integrity of white matter in terms of direction and rate of water diffusion, indicating altered timing of neural transmissions, thus disrupting integration of sensory information across multiple senses. "These are the tracts that are emblematic of someone with problems with sensory processing," said Dr. Pratik Mukherjee, senior author of the study (Bunim, 2013). "More frontal anterior white matter tracts are typically involved in children with only ADHD or autistic spectrum disorders. The abnormalities we found are focused in a different region of the brain, indicating SPD may be neuroanatomically distinct." Clearly further study is warranted to see if the findings generalize to females, different age groups, and those with varying intellectual capability.

In other studies, children diagnosed with SPD show increased electrodermal response and slower habituation to repeated sensory stimulation. The Sensory Challenge Protocol, used for a number of studies, is a laboratory procedure that measures physiological reactions to sensory stimulation. During this noninvasive procedure, children pretend they are astronauts and are hooked up to electrodes measuring electrodermal response, a commonly accepted index of sympathetic nervous system activity. They are then exposed to a series of 10 sensory stimuli in each of five sensory modalities: auditory (siren sounds), visual (blinking lights), olfactory (wintergreen oil), tactile (light touch by a feather on the chin), and vestibular (chair tipped back slowly) input (Miller, Reisman, McIntosh, & Simon, 2001). Each time the children diagnosed with SPD encountered sensory stimulation, they showed strong physiological reactions, whereas neurotypical children initially showed significant physiological reactions but soon became habituated, with minimal electrodermal response to subsequent stimulation.

A pilot study by Schaaf, Miller, Seawell, and O'Keefe (2003) looked specifically at the role of the parasympathetic nervous system using cardiac vagal tone, a widely accepted physiological index of stress. Here again, children with SPD showed physiological differences in terms of stress-related response as compared with their neurotypical counterparts.

Another study (Davies & Gavin, 2007) examined the relationship between brain function and SPD manifestations using EEG studies. This study found that kids with SPD demonstrated less sensory gating, which is the brain's mechanism for suppressing repeated or irrelevant stimuli. This study differentiated between the brain activity of typically developing children and those with SPD with 86 percent accuracy.

In all of these studies, it's as if the nervous system of the neurotypical child was saying, "Been there, done that . . . no big deal," while the nervous system of the child with sensory issues was saying, "Oh my, what is that?!" over and over and over. It's hard for most of us to imagine what it would be like to stay in a state of such high physiological arousal.

LIFE IS A MULTISENSORY EXPERIENCE

It's tempting to think of the sensory systems as distinct channels of input, yet the senses are interconnected. Each life experience affects more than one type of sensory receptor, and all stimuli are processed in the brain in many of the same structures.

Let's say you are sitting with your eyes closed, listening to music. The sound waves travel passively into your ears, stimulating auditory receptors in the cochlea in the inner ear. The vestibular apparatus, anatomically connected to the cochlea, is also stimulated through shared fluids and nerve fibers. At the same time, your tactile receptors pick up vibrations. The interoceptive system is impacted as well, with fast music shown to increase blood pressure, heart rate, and respiration and slow music shown to decrease heart rate and breathing frequency (Bernardi, Porta, & Sleight, 2006).

As you read about each sensory system in the following section and consider how difficulties with sensory skills impact the child you work with, remember that life is a multisensory experience and that each sensory system is intimately linked with the others.

Tactile Processing Issues

The child with tactile hypersensitivity finds many seemingly innocuous touch experiences threatening or difficult to tolerate. A pat on the back or getting his hair tousled may trigger protective reactions that, at their most extreme, tell the child to fight or flee. The hyposensitive or sensory-seeking child needs more input and tends to seek it out by touching people and objects excessively.

Difficulty With Dressing and Self-Care Tasks

The child may be very particular about clothing and take an unusually long time to find items that will feel okay for that day. This understandably causes stress and friction in the morning, putting the entire family on edge. He may peel off his clothes the moment he gets home at the end of the day and put on cozy sweatpants and a sweatshirt, putting the hood up and tucking his hands into the sleeves and pushing down in the pockets for deep pressure.

The child may prefer clothes to be tight for deep pressure or loose and nonbinding. The child may have a certain T-shirt she insists on wearing every day, sending a parent scrambling to do laundry each night. While the hypersensitive child may want her clothing just so, the hyposensitive child may not care much at all. She may not even notice that her shirt is inside out and her pants are twisted and unzipped.

Socks and shoes can be a problem too because they can hurt sensitive feet. A child may refuse to wear them and scream to wear flip-flops or Crocs even in cold weather because they don't hurt his feet. Another child may resist being barefoot because the feeling of the floor, carpet, grass, or sand is too difficult to bear. He may walk on tiptoes to have as little contact with surfaces as possible. A child may insist on wearing the same sneakers even though they are too small because she likes the compression. Winter boots can be a big problem too.

Self-care tasks like brushing teeth may be a nightmare because the bristles hurt the child's gums and the foam is too ticklish. The child may have a tantrum when it's time for hair washing, hair brushing, and haircuts because her scalp is so sensitive.

Getting Messy and Sticky

Children with tactile sensitivities may avoid touching materials that are difficult to interpret and hard to remove easily. They may resist art projects involving paint and glue or, if interested enough in the task, will become upset and want to wash their hands very frequently.

When a parent applies body lotion or sunblock, it may feel torturous. Such children may avoid playing in the sandbox and walking barefoot on grass or sand at the beach, but they may be willing to try these tactile experiences in a quiet location in which they are completely in control. So while a child may resist art activities in a room full of classmates, she might be delighted to do an art project at home or in therapy. Other kids are undersensitive and don't mind or don't notice getting messy or even crave it.

Picky Eating

Kids with tactile sensitivities usually have oral sensitivities—no surprise considering that the mouth is lined with skin. The tactile-defensive child may be highly selective about what food textures she will eat. Dry and crumbly, slippery, or mixed textures such as chunky soup may be intolerable. She may crave foods that are at a certain temperature.

Undersensitive eaters may also have difficulty at mealtime. They may crave strongly flavored foods with a lot of salt, sugar, or spices. They may tend to stuff their mouths to feel that something is in there and may not notice if they've pocketed food in their cheeks, both of which are potential choking hazards. They may prefer very cold or very hot foods, again because it gives them a lot of sensory cues. Kids with undersensitive mouths may also drool frequently because they are unaware of pooled saliva.

Socializing and Conformity

It can be heartbreaking for new parents to feel they cannot comfort their newborn who squirms away or arches her back when Mom or Dad attempts to hold her. Parent interactions at bath time, diapering, feeding, and other times may become very stressful for everyone involved.

Tactile defensiveness can amplify a gentle touch into something that is painful and upsetting. Children may set themselves apart as a coping mechanism, appearing to be aloof and uninterested. A boy may not feel comfortable in the jeans his classmates wear and a girl may not like the way the latest fashions feel and opt for clothing that is not in style.

Classmates become aware that Johnny is different; he doesn't join in team sports, won't engage in rough-and-tumble or messy play, avoids getting too close, and eats the same kind of sandwich every day. It's no fun being Johnny, and others can pick that up. Later on, dating and physical intimacy can become major challenges for adolescents and young adults.

The undersensitive or sensory-seeking child may have social problems too. He may stand too close to others, demand hugs and cuddles inappropriately, or be moving constantly, to the annoyance of teachers and classmates alike. Issues such as low muscle tone and motor incoordination may make the hyposensitive child clumsy on stairs and on the playground. Both sensory-seeking and hyposensitive children may struggle to stay still for extended periods and may instead be constantly on the move and fidgety, earning frequent redirection from the teacher and sometimes disdain from classmates. Other kids may shy away because the hyposensitive child does not follow social norms of behavior, sometimes unaware when his clothes are twisted, his hair is unkempt, or there is food on his face.

Temperature and Pain

Kids with tactile difficulties may be extremely sensitive to changes in temperature, taking a long time to adjust to changes in season or to going from the cold outdoors into a heated room, which makes transitions especially hard. Others are undersensitive to temperature and may need to be monitored carefully so they don't get burned or frostbitten.

There is a range in pain perception as well. Nancy Peske, coauthor of *Raising a Sensory Smart Child*, recalls how her son did not flinch and actually giggled when vaccinated, which indicated tactile undersensitivity (Biel & Peske, 2009). One child may collapse in tears at a paper cut while another doesn't even notice when her knees are scraped up and bloody after a fall on the playground.

Proprioceptive Processing Issues

The child who does not easily process input from the joints, muscles, and connective tissue struggles with body awareness, lacking the internal body maps we all use to guide us throughout our daily lives. Poor proprioception makes it difficult for the child to tell how much force she is using on toys and tools. When coloring she may press too hard and break her crayons, or, conversely, she may make such light marks that coloring is unsatisfying. When learning to write, she may rip the paper or constantly break her pencil point because she uses so much force. Excited to see Dad at the end of the day, she may give him such a hard hug that she practically knocks him over.

Space Cadets

The child with proprioceptive undersensitivity may be a "space cadet" because he doesn't know where his body parts are. He may be clumsy and have trouble navigating the classroom, bumping into furniture or tripping over classmates' feet. He may move awkwardly or slowly because he's not quite sure where his body parts are unless he looks. Both staying still and moving may require conscious effort. He may slide off his chair, trip on stairs, or stumble when he's walking or running because he's not getting good feedback from his lower body and trunk. At circle time he may lean against another child without realizing he is not sitting up straight, or he may sprawl out on the floor to get lots of body input. Kids with proprioceptive processing problems rely on vision to guide their movements. Put a blindfold on such a child when playing pin the tail on the donkey at a birthday party and she will be entirely unable to tell where she is.

Sensory Seeking

Proprioceptive sensory seekers may attempt to obtain more input in unacceptable ways, which may look like aggression or antisocial behavior. The kindergartner who stands in the corner throwing blocks during free play may be attempting to get needed input into the proprioceptors of his upper body rather than acting out. Behaviors such as kicking other people under the table, shoving classmates in line, and falling frequently on purpose may land the child in trouble since they seem like voluntary, attention-getting behaviors. They do, indeed, attract attention, but the intention is not to be annoying but instead to gain proprioceptive information for the child who doesn't quite know where his body ends and the rest of the world begins.

Socially, other children may avoid the proprioceptively challenged peer. Being clumsy, he may be the last one picked for team sports. He may be castigated for being too rough with others during sports and play activities. Or he may be shunned for being so spaced out.

Muscle Tone, Fatigue, and Alterations in Center of Gravity

Proprioceptors detect the stretch and pull on muscles and joints, sending a continuous stream of information to the brain for feedback about how much tension the muscles need at any given time. When this feedback loop is disrupted, the child may wind up with low muscle tone, or hypotonia. Muscle tone refers to the degree of tension when the muscle is not in use. Normal muscle tone is firm but not so much that it is hard to move. When a child has low muscle tone, the muscles seem loose and floppy and he lacks typical muscle power, resulting in rapid muscle fatigue and poor overall strength and endurance.

When a child has poor proprioception and difficulty telling where her body parts are in space relative to each other, it is difficult for her to tell whether she is sitting upright or standing up straight, resulting in poor seated and standing posture. The center of gravity may become skewed, so that the child seems to be walking with her weight tilted forward on the balls of her feet. When running, this child may appear to be always about to fall forward, and may often do so.

Developing Motor Skills

When most people learn new motor skills, they start by watching and monitoring their movements until they become automatic. When you tie your shoelaces, hopefully you don't have to watch each step to make sure you are doing it right. Your fingers know how to do it. A child learning to ride a bicycle may start off by looking at his feet and the handlebars rather than where he is going, until he figures out how to pump the pedals and steer.

When learning how to write, a child first visually analyzes the spatial relationships between horizontal, vertical, diagonal, and circular lines, watching every movement of her pencil until eventually she can write while focusing on a classroom lecture or on the content of her thoughts rather than individual letter strokes. The child with poor proprioception will continue to write slowly and effortfully, carefully forming each stroke, often with very poor legibility.

Self-Care and Feeding Problems

Getting dressed can be an arduous task as the child struggles to do buttons and snaps. Getting a shirt on and off may be tricky as well. Zippers, elastic waistbands, and loose-fitting shirts may be easiest for the child to handle.

Feeding can be a messy, time-consuming chore. The child may struggle to cut up his food or to pierce a piece of food with a fork. Spooning up thin liquids can be problematic since it's hard for the child to balance the food on the spoon and get it to the mouth without spilling. Thicker liquids such as yogurt and pudding may be easier. Reaching for a glass of milk may result in spills because the child has problems grading her force, frequently underreaching or overreaching for objects, especially if she has depth perception issues too.

Auditory Sensory Issues

As in all things sensory, people have a range of responses to auditory stimuli. Some are invigorated by intense, high-volume auditory input such as monster truck races and pounding rock-and-roll music. The faster and louder the better. Even if they do not have hearing loss (yet), some of these auditory stimulation seekers may speak at an unusually loud volume.

At the other end of the spectrum are people who react negatively to many if not most loud sounds and who greatly prefer gentle music with a slow, steady beat and quiet restaurants and activities.

Hearing involves more than just detecting sounds. Sound waves enter the ear passively, strike the eardrum, and are then converted to nerve impulses that are transmitted to the brain for analysis about where the sound originated from and whether it is important to attend to. If the neural messages are garbled along the way or misinterpreted in the brain, auditory processing is compromised. Excellent books on auditory processing disorders are available, including Teri James Bellis's (2003) *When the Brain Can't Hear*. This section addresses auditory sensitivity issues only.

A child may pass a hearing test with flying colors and yet have auditory problems. It may be that the child has difficulty processing sound volume or certain frequencies of sound (pitch), or that he struggles with active listening, which involves sorting through and processing what he hears.

While most of us begin to hear at zero to 15 decibels of sound, some can hear at zero or even negative decibels. Children with oversensitive hearing can actually hear too well, a condition called hyperacusis. Sounds that seem to be at normal volume may seem excessively loud to the hypersensitive person who may also perceive sounds others simply do not hear.

Further, certain high- or low-frequency sounds may be excruciatingly painful, described by Temple Grandin as like having a dentist drill hitting a nerve (Biel & Peske, 2009, p. xi). While it's normal for a newborn or young child to be startled and upset by loud, unexpected noises, most children become accustomed to common noises such as vacuum cleaners, hair dryers, blenders, flushing toilets, and even fire alarms. They may not enjoy the noise, but they no longer have dramatic reactions such as crying, screaming, or throwing tantrums. The hypersensitive child will usually continue to overreact well past the age when others outgrow such reactions.

Once a child has experienced a sound as painful and frightening, he may develop an aversion to it and may generalize his negative emotional reactions to environments and situations he feels have the potential to produce the same kinds of noxious experiences. While there is an emotional component, keep in mind that children may have true physiological hyperacusis as well as hypersensitivity to particular frequencies of sound. The sound does hurt their ears. This is something the child needs to be protected from through accommodations and acclimated to through an auditory sensory training program conducted by an OT. Learned negative behaviors related to the sound may also need to be addressed.

A hypersensitive child may detect and be distracted by sounds others don't seem to even hear. She may require absolute silence in the house in order to fall asleep and stay asleep. At school, she may hear her classmates in the back row as well as what's going on in the classroom next door. Music, typically classical music, played at low volume in a classroom with the aim of helping students focus or to help them nap may be perceived as abrasive and distracting.

Auditory Flooding

Kids with hyperacusis often have difficulty in noisy environments because there is so much sound to process. It's hard to tell where sounds are coming from. They struggle to filter out irrelevant sounds and to selectively attend to what is most important. This impacts their ability to attend and to learn and may result in off-task behaviors. It's very hard to listen to the teacher when other kids are talking in the room and the hallway, trucks are rumbling past, the heater is clanging, the fluorescent lights are buzzing, and a classmate is coughing. With so much to sort through in the sound field, a child may become easily distracted, tired, or overwhelmed.

Frequency Sensitivities

Children may also be sensitive to particular frequencies of sound. A low-frequency rumbling truck may be quite alarming, especially if the child has trouble locating where the truck is coming from and where it is likely to be going because, after all, if you can't localize a sound, primitive self-preservation instinct kicks in to protect yourself from approaching danger. Higher frequencies such as hair dryers can be very painful, as can squeaky, perky voices. Speech sounds have a range of frequencies. Lower-frequency sounds include *m*, *n*, and *b*, while *f*, *s*, and *th* are heard at higher frequencies.

Audiograms

Children with sensory issues, especially those with language delays, a history of ear infections, and negative responses to certain sounds, should have a comprehensive auditory examination by a qualified audiologist. School screenings typically use 35 decibels as the baseline to test for hearing loss (Eide & Eide, 2006) and do not use soundproofed rooms. To assess hyperacusis, testing for auditory thresholds should begin below zero decibels. Testing should occur in a soundproofed room. It's interesting to note that we can't achieve absolute zero decibels of noise. Even in a totally soundproofed, anechoic chamber, you would hear your own heartbeat and blood flowing—which some people with exquisitely sensitive hearing are actually able to hear in daily environments.

An audiogram will also test for sound detection thresholds at different frequencies. This is especially important when it comes to high and low frequencies of speech. Even a very mild hearing loss or oversensitivity to a specific frequency will affect the ability of the child to hear and process sounds at that frequency.

Functional Impact

A child with even very mild hearing impairment will miss out on certain sounds and information in the environment. If you've ever experienced clogged ears after an airplane ride or gotten water in your ears after swimming, you can imagine that this is not the time you would want to sit and listen to a teacher lecture or run around a noisy playground.

Children with auditory defensiveness may not wish to engage in many activities that most of their peers enjoy. Sensitive youngsters may become anxious and refuse to enter the room when taken to a "fun" toddler gym or music class because they are intimidated by all the commotion of other children plus noisy musical instruments or play equipment they do not know how to use.

The playground may be unendurable, with so much screeching, laughing, and talking sounds entering a child's ears from every direction, not to mention environmental noise such as cars and trucks. A child may prefer more sedentary options such as playing in the sandbox or playing quietly near a wall where sound is more contained and manageable.

Echoes in cavernous gymmasiums can make it difficult for the student to tolerate gym class or indoor athletics. Tiled bathrooms have lots of echoes because there is little sound-absorbing material. An auditory-sensitive child may become fearful of using public bathrooms, especially when the toilet has an auto-flush feature that appears to go off unpredictably, and automatic high-pitched hand dryers. It may help to teach the child to put a sticky note over the auto-flush sensor so it doesn't go off unexpectedly.

Sensitivities to the sounds of language may interfere with the development of receptive language as well as expressive language if certain sounds are not heard and processed well. Attending to teachers and parents may be difficult, especially when the language used is complex, multistep, and delivered in a tone of voice that is hard for the child to tolerate.

It may be impossible for a person with auditory sensitivities to maintain eye contact while you are speaking because it is simply too difficult to process two streams of sensory input at once, especially for those clients on the autistic spectrum or those with nonverbal learning disorder (NVLD). Watching your eyebrows move, trying to make sense of what the changes in your facial expression mean, and visual distortions may make following the content of what you are saying out of the question.

While some avoid eye contact, others may make constant eye contact, virtually boring holes into the other person's eyes. This too is problematic and off-putting to others. As normal maintenance of eye contact is a basic social skill, the child who cannot process sight and sound simultaneously has an added obstacle to socializing.

Some people who struggle to process sounds hyperfocus on what they are doing by "turning off" their ears. Blocking out ambient noise by focusing on one thing to the exclusion of all else is a hard-earned skill that then makes it difficult to shift attention from one thing to another. A parent or teacher may become frustrated and annoyed when he or she calls the child's name and the child does not respond. While we are used to seeing this with kids who are watching a favorite TV show or playing a video game, it's less obvious when the child is engaged in something quiet such as building with blocks, reading, or coloring. It's a sensory-driven attention shift problem rather than preference or rudeness.

Visual Processing Issues

When you consider vision, chances are you think about visual acuity and whether a child can see 20/20. Her eyes do indeed need to accurately detect visual stimuli, but, just as importantly, her brain must be able to remember what she sees, process what it means, and determine the best response. Furthermore, ocular-motor, visual attention, and visual sensitivity issues can interfere with function, even for a child with perfect vision.

Ocular-Motor and Eye-Teaming Skills

The eye muscles need to keep the eyes aligned and moving smoothly and simultaneously, with the eyes working together like a pair of binoculars, melding the two fields of vision into one clear visual field. Many children with sensory challenges have both ocular-motor and eye-teaming skill problems, especially those with low muscle tone in other parts of their body. A child may struggle with visual issues such as convergence insufficiency, which makes it hard for the eyes to work together, resulting in blurred or double vision and eye fatigue, especially for prolonged close-up tasks. Another issue may be strabismus, in which the eyes have a neuromuscular misalignment and are unable to fuse the images from two eyes into one.

Such visual problems make it hard or even impossible for the child to:

- Maintain visual clarity, especially for sustained close work such as reading, writing, and stringing beads.
- Make smooth saccadic eye movements to scan items in an organized way, such as when reading across lines of print.
- Follow a moving object, such as a ball in order to catch it or to keep sight of the teacher walking around the room.
- Perceive depth, such as the distance between the child's body and items in the environment such as a ball as it approaches.
- Keep the visual field fixed while moving, such as keeping the playground visually stable when you run.
- Refocus from near to far and back again, such as when taking notes from the board.
- Discriminate between foreground and background to identify a particular object or person in a busy visual field, such as a sock in a drawer or a parent in a store.

When vision is not accurate, stable, and dependable, simple tasks like looking into someone's eyes, climbing stairs, navigating obstacles, reading, writing, and playing are difficult. Visual stimuli such as birds flying in the sky or kids running can be upsetting for a child whose visual field is not reliable. Difficulties with depth perception make ball play frustrating and descending stairs spooky since the child cannot tell the distance to the next step.

With visual distortions, printed letters, people, and objects in the environment may appear unstable, blurring, moving, or changing, or may disappear and reappear. A parent's face may look very strange when she knits her eyebrows, floor tiles and steps may seem to shift, and so on. Understandably, the child might prefer to avoid eye contact, avoid climbing stairs, and remain relatively sedentary. Spinning wheels on a car or lining up toys may be preferable. Some children may rely on their peripheral vision since doing so reduces or eliminates the distortions in the central part of their vision. The child who turns her head away from you may actually be using her best field of vision to see you.

If there are concerns about a child's vision skills, or if he is struggling with reading or other vision-related tasks, it is essential that the child receive a comprehensive vision examination by a qualified vision care professional such as a developmental optometrist or pediatric ophthalmologist. Please see Chapter 5 for more on vision care specialists.

Visual Attention

A child's world is crammed full of constant visual images. As with other types of sensory input, as children mature, ideally they learn how to filter out irrelevant sensory stimuli in order to focus on what's important to attend to. If a child struggles with sensory gating and filtering, he can easily become overstimulated because he attends to every visual cue. In a classroom, the child may be so busy looking at everybody and everything on the walls that he misses out on important visual cues from the teacher and appears to be inattentive.

Kids with hyperopia (farsightedness) are often misdiagnosed with attention issues because it is physically difficult for them to focus on the work at hand. Further, if overwhelmed by visual images or vision issues such as convergence insufficiency, some kids simply defocus and zone out. They may be hard to engage, preferring to daydream or engage in self-absorbed activity. Other children visually hyperfocus. For example, a child may become so involved in watching TV that he truly does not hear a parent calling for him to sit down for dinner. It's not that he is ignoring the parent or doesn't want to "be good" but that he struggles with shifting his attention away from what he is doing onto a new incoming sensory stimulus.

Visually, most of us focus on the big picture and then sort through the visual details. Many people, especially those on the autism spectrum or with learning disabilities, focus on the details instead. It may be difficult to see the forest because the individual leaves on each tree are so visually appealing.

Many children crave visual input, staring at shiny objects, spinning wheels on a toy car, or letters of the alphabet. They may have large collections of objects, almost to the point of hoarding. These visuals are predictable and safe, and looking at them may feel like a safe escape from a world that is visually overwhelming. Children who seemed fixated on numbers or letters may seem to be perseverating in a nonpurposeful activity but are often early writers and readers.

Visual Sensitivity Issues

Some people are hypersensitive to light, contrast, color, and patterns. At its most severe, usually for people on the autistic spectrum, visual hypersensitivity may feel like old-fashioned TV station static or may result in temporary visual whiteouts. Issues include:

- Light sensitivity. Bright lights, sunlight, and glare may assault the nervous system and result in physical discomfort, fatigue, dizziness, anxiety, headaches, and other problems. Fluorescent lighting is particularly problematic as sensitive people can see and hear it pulse on and off. Downcast lighting can also be quite uncomfortable. Looking into a computer screen for long periods may cause eyestrain and headaches.

- Contrast sensitivity. Some people have difficulty differentiating between light and dark. Contrast sensitivity issues make it hard to read or to navigate safely through space on a bicycle or to drive. Most people have no problem reading black type on a white page. In cases of low contrast sensitivity, letters will appear faded and hard to see. Loss of contrast sensitivity is usually a sign of eye disease. Some people with hypersensitivity find the contrast too strong and intense to look at for long. When the letters appear too dark, for example, it may be hard to look at black type against white paper. Print resolution may also be impaired, meaning that letters appear to move, shimmer, or break apart. Difficulties with contrast and print resolution become more marked as a child matures and reads increasingly smaller print with more letters and words per page and is expected to read for longer periods. Often people with contrast sensitivity issues will do well with colored overlays that alter the dark-to-light ratio.

• Color and pattern sensitivity. Lots of kids have strong color preferences, classically pink and purple for girls and blue and green for boys despite efforts to avoid gender stereotyping. Some kids with SPD simply cannot tolerate certain colors. A child may freak out in a bright yellow room, for example, because the color is unacceptable to his visual system. An undersensitive child may require bright colors and even flashing lights to draw her attention to a toy.

Remember that vision and motor skills are interconnected. We use our eyes to guide us through most new movement patterns. When learning to write, a child uses her vision to guide each stroke. Some of us continue to use our vision when typing on a keyboard if we have not learned to touch type, which relies on our proprioceptive sense for finger placement. When learning to roller skate, a child may watch his feet at first. As these movement patterns become more familiar, mental maps become hard-wired, and the child relies less on vision. Instead there is greater reliance on internalized motor plans as the vestibular and proprioceptive senses take over.

Vestibular Processing Issues

As noted in Chapter 1, the vestibular system is located in the inner ear, detecting changes in gravitational forces and head position. When the vestibular system is working efficiently, it is the primary organizer of sensory input, helping you balance and visually orient yourself as you move through space. The vestibular system also plays a key role in attention and alertness. The central nervous system processes vestibular and other sensory input by assessing for potential threat and then responding accordingly: facilitating protective responses if appropriate ("danger—watch out!"), inhibiting protective responses ("nothing to worry about here"), or modulating protective responses ("not sure—proceed with caution"). This assessment can be out of whack for the child with a vestibular system that is functioning poorly.

The child with vestibular problems may have low muscle tone because the messages telling the muscles how much to contract are not getting through. When the child attempts to move, he may not be able to activate his muscles in an appropriate way, interfering with balance and muscle coordination. As a result, he may tend to avoid movement activities he perceives as challenging or scary.

Such a child may not be able to accurately interpret how her head and body are oriented in order to maintain equilibrium and balance. She may feel understandably unsafe and insecure when moving because she can't tell which way is up and where she is going. Changes in head position may be disorienting and she may avoid lifting her feet from the ground. She may become dizzy very easily or never at all. The visual field may be unstable as she moves; for example, when she rides a merry-go-round the entire world seems to be spinning along with her.

When a child with vestibular issues rides in a car or an airplane, the vestibular system senses motion while the visual system does not, and these mixed signals can result in motion sickness. Yet others may fall asleep the minute the vehicle starts moving. For some babies, getting vestibular input through rocking, being pushed in a stroller, or riding in a car may be the only way they can fall asleep.

Other kids may be agile, moving constantly, fidgeting and squirming, and sometimes taking excessive risks like climbing too high and biking too fast without monitoring traffic. Because of their difficulty inhibiting their need for movement, they may annoy others, miss out on vital learning opportunities, and be prone to injuries.

Gravitational Insecurity

The child with gravitational insecurity reacts to changes in head position or movement disproportionately to the actual risk. The child feels unable to maintain his balance against the force of gravity. This may be due to poor integration of vestibular and cerebellar functions, primarily difficulty processing information from the utricle and the saccule (Fisher & Bundy, 1989; May-Benson & Koomar, 2007).

Symptoms include fear of falling, being upside down as when hanging on monkey bars, or having feet leave the ground as in a somersault. Walking on a bumpy or pliant surface such as a rocky path or in snow or sand may be distressing, as can stepping from one kind of surface to another, such as from a concrete sidewalk onto a grassy area. Traveling in a car, riding a bicycle, skating, or other movement challenge may be upsetting, as can something as innocuous as bending over to pick up a fallen object or to tie shoes (the child will soon learn to pick up the object by bending at the hips and knees but keeping his head upright, or to put her foot up on a chair to tie her laces).

The gravitationally insecure child tends to opt for sedentary activities such as reading, arts and crafts, or building things, avoiding active physical play. The child may abhor having his feet off the floor, refusing to go on swings or do a somersault. He may prefer to stay low to the ground where he is most secure. He may be willing to challenge himself physically, but only if he is in control. He may become fearful and upset if movement is forced upon him, fussing when placed on a diaper changing table as a baby, crying when put into an infant swing, and avoiding rough play and team sports when he is older.

Oversensitivity to Movement

Kids with vestibular overreactivity may be uncomfortable, anxious, or quite intolerant of fast movement or spinning. They may get dizzy or nauseated easily, especially when riding in a car, using playground equipment, or on amusement park rides. Just looking at someone else on a roller coaster may make the child dizzy or nauseated because it triggers a vestibular-ocular reflex.

Hyposensitivity to Movement and Sensory Seeking

When a child underresponds to vestibular input, she may be appear to be somewhat lazy and loose-limbed, like a floppy rag doll, as she struggles to work against gravity. Transitioning from one position to another, such as getting up off the couch in order to walk, may be effortful, and she may avoid play such as running and athletics. She may actually move a lot but not necessarily in an organized, smooth way.

The child who actively seeks out movement input is quite another story. This child may be in constant motion, again because his vestibular system works so poorly. He may feel right only when on the go, running wildly in the playground, rocking in his seat, walking in circles or around the perimeter of the room, bouncing a ball, or fidgeting with objects in order to meet his body's intense craving for input. When he is older, he will ideally channel this into a healthy outlet such as soccer or track or may continue to engage in disorganized sensory seeking such as driving too fast, with the need for movement so compelling that safety may be compromised.

Smell Processing Issues

As noted earlier, the olfactory (smell) system is a primitive sense that alerts us to danger in the environment such as spoiled food, smoke, and many toxic fumes. Throughout the day, odor molecules travel along free-flowing air currents into the nose. When we want to smell more of something, we sniff to pull more of these molecules into our nasal cavities where chemical receptors send an impulse up the olfactory tract. Unlike all other sensory information, only the olfactory sense sends messages directly to the limbic system of the brain, instantaneously triggering emotions and memories.

When you think of smell you may think of roses, apple pie, or your stinky dog. Absolutely everything and everyone has an odor, which most of us learn to block out unless it is particularly fragrant or repugnant.

Smell Oversensitivity

The child with overreactive olfactory processing may experience a continuous barrage of smells and have strong responses to smells most others enjoy, notice but tolerate, or may not even be consciously aware of. The smell of other people's bodies and breath plus any perfumes or lotions may nauseate a sensitive child. Certain food aromas may make the child gag. The child may be very sensitive to the smell of cleaning products, body care products, and the off-gassing of new carpeting and furniture. Supermarkets, restaurants, and holiday gatherings where there are many food smells and lots of people with various aromas may be hard for this child to tolerate. Between the varied cleanliness of classmates, smelly locker rooms and socks in gym class, assorted foods and open garbage bins for emptying trays in the cafeteria, plus strong cleaning products, school can be especially unpleasant. Indoor swimming pools, zoos, and gas stations can be hellish for a sensitive nose. Smell sensitivity tends to increase when a person has a migraine headache.

Smell Undersensitivity and Sensory Seeking

Some people are undersensitive to smell. They do not pick up aromas easily and may have a decreased appetite. Because they may not notice strong smells such as smoke, safety may be an issue. In rare cases, hyposmia or anosmia, reduced or total inability to perceive smell, may occur due to cranial nerve injury, respiratory infections, head trauma, certain medications, and other conditions.

Because they smell so poorly, smell-undersensitive kids may sniff things as a means of exploration or stimulation. A child may smell her pencil before using it, a book while she is reading it, or an animal while petting it. More oddly, some may sniff other people in order to pick up their scent more strongly. This is seen most often in children with cognitive disabilities or autism spectrum disorders (ASDs), as there is a higher prevalence of smell underreactivity.

Some children actively seek out very strong odors in inappropriate ways. For example, a teen with an intellectual disability who lived in a group home would run to sniff garbage cans whenever possible and would, if not prevented, roll around the lawn if it had been recently fertilized. This boy learned to get the olfactory input he craved by putting Vicks VapoRub around his nostrils before going on group walks. Less intense essential oils may be used in much the same way to preempt and satisfy overstimulating or unacceptable smell needs.

Taste (Gustatory) Processing Issues

Many toddlers are picky eaters, reducing the number and kinds of foods they will eat as their taste buds mature. However, the child with taste and other sensitivities tends to be an exceptionally picky eater, eating an extremely limited number of foods due to difficulties with taste, texture, temperature, smell, jaw strength, and other factors (see Chapter 6).

A child who is oversensitive to tastes may insist on a very bland diet consisting mostly of pasta, macaroni and cheese, and chicken nuggets. Once the taste-sensitive person finds something that tastes okay, he may always request the same thing meal after meal and become upset when his preferred food is not available or is prepared in a different way.

The child who is undersensitive may crave strongly flavored foods, squeezing lemon onto his fish sticks, pouring hot sauce onto his burger, and dumping salt and pepper onto his French fries.

Alterations in taste (and smell) can be a sign of zinc deficiency. An extreme zinc deficiency can lead to a complete loss of appetite, contributing to a later diagnosis of anorexia (Lask, Fosson, Rolfe, & Thomas, 1993). In a case of extreme food cravings and aversions, zinc levels should be assessed by a doctor or nutritionist through a blood test rather than relying on fun but not 100 percent reliable do-it-yourself taste tests such as Zinc Tally.

COMORBID CONDITIONS

SPD casts a wide net, affecting kids, teens, and adults with a variety of diagnoses as well as those who do not meet any other diagnostic criteria. In cases in which the child does have a concurrent diagnosis such as autism, ADHD, or anxiety, addressing any sensory processing challenges can dramatically reduce some of the most marked traits of the diagnosis.

Autism Spectrum Disorders

ASDs are clinically defined by impairments in social interaction, verbal and nonverbal communication, and stereotyped, repetitive, inflexible behavior and restricted interests. Within the diagnosis there is a wide range of cognitive ability, language development, and daily life function. There are many known etiologies including genetic variations such as fragile X, environmental exposures such as in utero valproic acid exposure, and prematurity (Marco, Hinkley, Hill, & Nagarajan, 2011; Schneider & Przewłocki, 2005). Other contributing factors under study include exposure to environmental toxins such as heavy metals like mercury as well as having an older father.

While not everyone with sensory processing issues has autism, almost all people with autism do have sensory processing issues–some of the most dramatic and disabling ones. Over 90 percent of children with autism have sensory abnormalities, with symptoms in multiple sensory domains (Leekam, Nieto, Libby, Wing, & Gould, 2007). A study by Dr. Stanley Greenspan and Dr. Serena Wieder (1997) found that 94 percent had sensory issues, including underreactivities, overreactivities, and mixed reactivity to a variety of sensory input and that 100 percent had auditory processing dysfunction and motor planning problems.

Interestingly, children with autism appear to have a lower baseline arousal level. A 2009 study compared sensory processing difficulties in children with ASD as well as children diagnosed with SPD alone (Schoen, Miller, Brett-Green, & Nielsen, 2009). Sympathetic nervous system arousal and reactivity were measured across five sensory domains using the Sensory Challenge Protocol described earlier in this chapter. Results showed, unsurprisingly, that kids with ASD and SPD had significantly more noteworthy sensory-related behaviors than typically developing children. Remarkably, though, children with ASD had lower baseline physiological arousal, and reactivity after each sensory stimulus was higher in children with SPD but not ASD, especially to the first trial of each sensory stimulus. The kids with ASD had greater vestibular and proprioceptive underreactivity and greater taste and smell overreactivity. Overall, the SPD group had more atypical sensory-seeking behavior than the children on the autistic spectrum.

A more recent study found that children with autism are extremely sensitive to motion, seeing visual stimuli twice as quickly as neurotypical children of the same age (Foss-Feig, Tadin, Schauder, & Cascio, 2013).

What are the clinical implications? While sensory hypersensitivities and hyposensitivities are not unique to kids with autism, they tend to be most significant and thus potentially disabling in this population. Atypical sensory processing is directly related to the unusual behavioral responses typically observed in children with ASDs, ranging from withdrawal to self-injurious behavior in those unable to communicate their extreme discomfort. And while children with autism are typically strong visual learners found to excel at perceiving patterns and attending to details, visual sensitivity to movement may lead to sensory overstimulation as children on the spectrum interact in busy environments. Furthermore, watching the subtle movements that create changes in facial expressions as others speak may further aggravate language processing difficulties.

Attention Deficits

Imagine 10-year-old Jackson as he sits at the dinner table with his family. While everyone is waiting nicely as Mom serves the food, Jackson rocks back and forth in his chair and kicks his little sister, who whines that her big brother is hurting her. "I didn't mean to do it," Jackson says, and makes an effort to keep away from her, banging his feet into the table legs instead. "Will you please sit still?" Dad says.

Oh gosh, it's chicken and rice for dinner. It's dry and stringy and gets stuck in his throat and makes him want to gag. "This is going to be bad," he thinks, and starts tapping his spoon on his plate to keep his mind off the last time he had chicken and nearly vomited. "Stop that immediately," says Mom. "You know I hate this barfy food. Why can't we have burgers?" he responds. He reaches for his milk and spills it on the floor. Smarty the dog comes to the rescue to lick it up. He has kibble breath. Jackson smacks Smarty on the head and he nips at Jackson. "Why did you hit Smarty so hard, Jackson? He did nothing! Go to your room. Right. Now." Jackson is confused because all he did was pet his dog, whom he loves despite his breath, and he's mad because he is hungry too. "I hate you!" he yells as he stomps off to his room.

What is happening here to Jackson and his family? He shows symptoms of inattention, hyperactivity, and impulsivity. A child like Jackson may appear to have a straightforward case of ADHD yet something else might actually be going on. When he couldn't sit still in his chair, rocking and kicking, was he hyperactive or seeking out sensory stimulation his body needed? Did he spill his milk because he wasn't paying attention or because he had difficulty coordinating his eyes and hands? Did he kick his sister and hit his dog because he was impulsive or because he could not use proprioceptive input to fine-tune his movements? Were all of these increased symptoms a result of food smells and textures he could not tolerate?

A child may have ADHD, SPD, or, as is frequently the case, both. In so many ways these are lookalike diagnoses since many kids with sensory challenges struggle with issues such as being easily distracted by conflicting stimuli and being constantly moving or fidgety due to low muscle tone, poor body awareness, and vestibular problems. It's incredibly hard for a student to focus on what the teacher is saying when he has auditory processing issues, is distracted by the visual clutter in the room and the flickering overhead fluorescent lights, and can't stop thinking about how itchy his socks are. When a child on the playground is running in circles, bumping and crashing into kids, swinging on the swings and not letting others have a turn, that child may be seeking out vestibular and proprioceptive input to help his nervous system feel better.

Studies are starting to clarify the neurological differences between ADHD and SPD. A study by Miller, Nielson, and Schoen (2012) compared children with clinical ADHD, the sensory modulation disorder subtype of SPD, and those diagnosed with both to consider whether ADHD and SPD are, indeed distinct conditions. The study found that both groups had significantly more sensory, attention, motor activity, impulsivity, and emotional challenges than neurotypical kids. It found that the ADHD group had more inattention than the SPD group. The dually diagnosed group had more sensory-related behaviors than purely ADHD kids and more attention problems than purely SPD kids. The SPD group had more sensory issues, more somatic complaints, anxiety, depression, and difficulty adapting than ADHD kids, as well as greater physiological (electrodermal) reactivity to sensory stimuli than the ADHD group and neurotypical kids. There is, indeed, a difference.

It's well known that issues such as learning disabilities, cognitive delays, or simply a poor match between a student's abilities and academic demands can cause restless behavior at school that looks similar to ADHD, per the *DSM-IV Training Guide* (Rapoport & Ismond, 1996). Clearly, sensory processing issues also need to be considered. Child psychiatrist Dr. Larry Silvers, author of *The Misunderstood Child*, asserts that ADHD is actually the least common reason for hyperactivity, inattention, distractibility, and impulsivity, while the leading reasons are anxiety, depression, learning disability, and SPD (Silver, 1998, p. 77). All of these factors need to be taken into account when helping the client with attention challenges.

OTHER PSYCHIATRIC CONDITIONS

Sensory processing problems can affect kids, teens, and adults with a wide range of diagnoses—from anxiety to depression to bipolar to obsessive-compulsive disorder to oppositional defiant disorder. While some children do indeed have psychiatric disorders alone, symptoms may sometimes actually be strong behavioral responses to sensory events. Kids may be tense and anxious, anticipating the next awful occurrence, or withdrawn and sad because they are in such a low state of nervous system arousal. Some kids get frustrated by being at the mercy of their senses and act out in inappropriate ways. When disorders—psychiatric and sensory—do actually co-occur, psychiatric symptoms will be significantly reduced when the sensory issues are addressed.

The hypersensitive child who becomes overaroused at a crowded, noisy birthday party is doing so because the stimulation is intolerable, not necessarily because she has an anxiety disorder. When the offending stimulation is removed, the anxious behavior should go away. Unfortunately, as children develop, they begin to notice that they are different and that what bothers them simply is not an issue for most other people. They also worry about facing similar situations. The child who has low energy, draped over a couch like a wet noodle due to underreactivity, is not necessarily clinically depressed. Sensory overresponsivity in particular has been linked to social-emotional problems, anxiety, and depression (Kinnealy & Fuiek, 1999).

SPD behaviors are always related to a sensory challenge, at least initially. Children with sensory issues can appear to be moody because their reactions to sensory stimuli are so intense and it takes a long time to recover. It may be hard for parents to figure out what is going to set the child off, and they may complain of feeling like they are walking on eggshells.

Kids with SPD have good days when they feel great and navigate sensory experiences optimally as well as bad days ruined by intolerable sensory events. However, the mood cycling seen in bipolar disorder is not seen in SPD, although the child may have both diagnoses.

Kids who feel that the world is an unpredictable place full of uncontrollable sights, sounds, smells, and more may develop some personal rituals and rigid behavior to cope. A child may insist on having a super-organized bedroom with books in size order on the shelves or may insist on washing his hands the moment they get dirty. Attempts to bring overwhelming visual stimuli under control and to cope with the unbearable sensation of messy hands is far different from the obsessive, persistent thoughts, impulses, or images that lead to the repetitive behaviors or mental acts that are hallmarks of obsessive-compulsive disorder.

The child who overreacts to stimulation and shows out-of-bounds behavior when forced into intolerable situations may act out in extreme ways to cope with or escape the sensory insult. Extreme act-ing-out behaviors may land the child with a diagnosis of oppositional defiant disorder, but the diagnosis may not be appropriate if insuffer-able sensory stimulation is triggering the behavior.

Fragile X syndrome symptoms range from mild learning disabili-ties to significant intellectual disability with overreactivity to sensory stimuli, hyperactivity, anxiety and mood instability, and other symp-toms. Diagnosed through genetic testing, fragile X is the most com-mon form of inherited intellectual disability in boys, and is generally milder in girls.

Even when a psychiatric diagnosis is crystal clear, it's essential to assess for sensory issues that may aggravate symptoms. Sensory problems have been noted in a variety of disorders such as Tourette's syndrome (TS). People with Tourette's frequently have tactile sensi-tivities, auditory processing problems, poor balance and coordination, and other issues. The person with Tourette's who is able to suppress motor and vocal tics most of the time may become unable to do so in the face of overwhelming sensory demands.

In recent years, there has been a renewed interest in the role of sensory function in schizophrenia, including the sensory distortions experienced by those with early schizophrenic symptoms (Javitt, 2009). Research into triggers for full-blown symptoms finds that peo-ple with high-functioning schizophrenia report that exercising, eating a healthy diet, avoiding alcohol, getting adequate sleep, and control-ling sensory input are key strategies (Saks, 2013). For many, this requires reducing sensory input, such as keeping living space mini-mally stimulating with bare walls, no TV, and quiet music, or using sensory modalities to self-regulate such as playing distracting or loud music to mask other sounds (Saks, 2013). Using sensory input to self-regulate is discussed in Chapter 4.

Cerebral Palsy, Down Syndrome, and Other Disabilities

Children with Down syndrome typically have low muscle tone, joint hypermobility, poor motor skills, sensory hyper- or hyposensitivities, poor sensory discrimination skills, and many other issues.

Children born with torticollis, a twisting of the neck that tips the head to one side, have limited range of motion in the neck, neck pain, and other symptoms. An active stretching and strengthening program is in order at a very young age to avoid significant limitations in vision and to build tolerance for tactile input in affected areas.

Children who receive tube feedings due to conditions such as Hirschsprung disease, digestive disorders, inability to swallow or unsafe swallowing, failure to thrive, and other issues may develop oral motor defensiveness. If and when they become able to eat by mouth, they may not be able to tolerate a wide variety of food textures and flavors.

Children with physical disabilities such as cerebral palsy and hemiplegia typically have sensory processing difficulties on two fronts, with degree of impact depending on the location and severity of the damage. First, the disabling condition may have damaged physiological structures and thus the ability to pick up incoming sensory input. Second, mobility restrictions may limit access to sensory stimulation.

The child with limited mobility may not have typical opportunities to move through space and challenge gravity. A child with cerebral palsy, for example, may have muscle tightness and joint contractures that make it difficult to move and interfere with accessing tactile, vestibular, and proprioceptive input. Cranial nerve palsies, strabismus, and nystagmus may make it difficult for the child to integrate and use visual and vestibular input.

Special care should be taken to minimize excess sensory-based disability by providing well-thought-out sensory stimulation. For the child who uses a wheelchair, this means regularly getting out of that chair and onto the floor or into a stander to promote weight-bearing through the joints as well as to provide sensory simulation to various parts of the body.

Learning Differences

Kids with learning disabilities and giftedness both appear to have an increased incidence of sensory issues. For the learning disabled or developmentally delayed child, poor visual processing may make it hard to maintain visual attention and to learn to read and complete worksheets and bubble sheet tests, while auditory issues may interfere with following directions and what is being taught. Poor integration of sensory input makes it hard for a child to maintain the optimal state of arousal necessary to listen, learn, and thrive.

Meanwhile, gifted and profoundly gifted have long been recognized to have increased sensitivities, referred to as "overexcitabilities," that is, inborn, heightened psychological and nervous system sensitivity, awareness, and intensity. A study shows that the gifted population does, indeed, have greater sensitivity to their environment and reacts with heightened emotional and behavioral responses compared with children of average intelligence (Gere, Capps, Mitchell, & Grubbs, 2009). These overexcitabilities or heightened sensitivities likely contribute to exceptional creativity and intelligence and are not considered problematic unless they interfere with the child's ability to engage in activities and tasks that are meaningful to the child and the family.

RISK FACTORS FOR SPD

Sensory processing difficulties cast a wide net, but have increased prevalence in children who have had experiences that negatively impacted their brain function and thus have interfered with the development of a well-functioning, smoothly integrated nervous system.

Genetics

While no specific genetic markers for SPD have been identified, it does appear to have a genetic component. Many of the conditions that predispose kids to sensory issues such as autism, Down syndrome, and fragile X syndrome do have a genetic basis. One or both parents may have sensory processing issues themselves. Siblings—especially twins—often have sensory problems too.

Prematurity

Babies born prematurely have a greatly increased risk for sensory problems, especially those born earliest and tiniest. The premature baby's nervous system has not matured enough to handle the intense sensory input of the world outside the warm, cozy womb. Newborn intensive care units do their best to nurture preemies but cannot prevent inevitable exposures to bright lights and beeping equipment, needle sticks, and other noxious sensory input.

Many, but not all, preemies tend to:

- Be highly sensitive to noise, light, touch, and movement beyond their second birthday.
- Develop oral defensiveness secondary to unpleasant oral input from feeding tubes, respirators, and suctioning which interferes with feeding.
- Be either distractible and active or quieter and sleepier than is typical.
- Be at risk for vision problems such as nearsightedness and poor binocularity.
- Retain startle reflexes beyond typical age.
- Have abnormal muscle tone, that is, high tone with resulting stiffness, low tone with resulting floppiness, or a mix of both. While muscle tone problems may be a serious, permanent neurological symptom, in preemies it may be a temporary condition that resolves by around 18 months of age.

Birth Trauma, Frequent Illnesses, and Hospitalizations

Oxygen deprivation, cesarean delivery, neonatal surgeries, and other medical procedures increase the baby's risk of sensory problems. For example, painful stimuli to fragile skin from needle sticks, IV lines, and bandages may result in tactile defensiveness, while tube feedings for extended periods may lead to oral defensiveness. Medically fragile and frequently hospitalized children unfortunately may be deprived of adequate sensory stimulation at critical times necessary for neurological development, especially if prolonged bed rest is required.

Exposure to Toxins

Fetal exposure to drugs, alcohol, tobacco, and heavy metals such as lead and mercury greatly increase the risk for a host of problems. For example, while physical disabilities occur in 25–30 percent of infants exposed prenatally to cocaine or methamphetamine, neurobehavioral difficulties are even more common and include difficulties with sensory overload and self-regulation (Chasnoff, 2010). Babies exposed to alcohol in utero may develop alcohol-related neurobehavioral defects including cognitive problems, growth deficiencies, and central nervous system issues. Sensory issues in children with fetal alcohol syndrome or its milder manifestations include sensory hypersensitivity and auditory processing deficits. Heavy metal poisoning causes many neurological problems, including severe brain injury, motor incoordination, learning disabilities, behavioral problems, damage to sensory receptors, and significant sensory processing difficulties.

Adoption

Children who have been adopted are at increased risk, especially those adopted from overseas orphanages. The child adopted from an overseas institutional setting may have been born prematurely or at a low birth weight along with other issues due to poor nutrition, limited or no access to prenatal care, or exposure to toxins such as lead, alcohol, and drugs. These factors are then compounded by the environment in some orphanages, which, sadly, do not always provide adequate sensory stimulation and loving attention to vulnerable babies. Babies may be bottle propped, swaddled for excessive periods, rarely held, and given inadequate opportunities for movement and sensory exploration. This is certainly not the case for all overseas orphanages, but when such sensory deprivation does occur, children adopted into new loving homes can struggle with significant sensory challenges as they adjust to new, highly stimulating environments with unfamiliar sights, sounds, touches, and so on. Domestic adoptions of children who have lived in group homes and in foster care present a lower degree of risk due to better living conditions for the children, with more typical opportunities for sensory stimulation as well as greater likelihood of prenatal care.

Food and Environmental Sensitivities

People with SPD often have symptoms that wax and wane, which is why keeping a behavior journal is so important (see Chapter 6). While symptom expression depends on several variables including whether the child is well rested, the quality of food eaten and resulting nutritional status, emotional and physical stressors, and the intensity and duration of sensory processing demands, some families find that their child is worse off at a certain time of year. In the spring, hay fever can make for a very uncomfortable child with heightened sensory issues due to factors such as ear congestion and histamine-driven skin sensitivity. In autumn, wet leaves can lead to mold growth, which some people are quite sensitive to. Pollution, harsh cleaning products, and more can also wreak havoc with a sensitive nervous system (see Chapter 6 for helpful strategies).

Kids with sensory issues who also are intolerant or outright allergic to particular foods often find their sensory symptoms greatly improved when the food is removed from the diet. Gluten—a protein found in wheat, barley, rye, and other grains—increasingly appears to be an especially pervasive culprit, especially as very refined gluten products now dominate many children's diets in the form of bread, pasta, muffins, and so on. Gluten intolerance (which in effect is similar to celiac disease, an autoimmune disorder) can result in symptoms including indigestion, fatigue, headaches, skin itchiness, moodiness, gastrointestinal distress, and disturbed sleep. Some kids with sensory and behavioral issues feel and function much better when most or all gluten is eliminated. Many children also show improvements when lactose—the sugar found in milk and other dairy products—is removed from the diet. It is worth examining the client's diet, especially if he is an extremely picky eater or has frequent gastrointestinal problems such as gas, bloating, diarrhea, or constipation. Collaborating with a nutritionist is recommended (see Chapter 5).

DIAGNOSING SPD

More and more pediatricians are becoming aware of SPD and how sensory issues are affecting their patients and families. Nevertheless, a significant number remain who are not familiar with sensory processing difficulties. All too many parents find that when they report their observations and concerns, they are simply told to wait and see or, worse yet, are patronized as nervous new parents. As the baby misses key developmental milestones—often not crawling or walking, eating solids, or speaking on time—they are eventually referred to early intervention and an astute early childhood specialist who, hopefully, picks up on the sensory problems.

Professionals on the front lines in the clinic, in children's homes, and in schools have long been aware of sensory problems. OTs, developmental pediatricians, and some savvy clinicians have become increasingly aware of and able to recognize sensory processing problems, though the term is only now becoming as familiar as some of the other alphabet soup diagnoses like ADHD.

Zero to Three's *Diagnostic Classification of Mental Health and Developmental Disorders of Infancy and Early Childhood* has included "Sensory Processing Disorders of Regulation" for infants and toddlers for quite some time (Zero to Three, 2005). The Interdisciplinary Council on Developmental and Learning Disabilities, founded by the late psychiatrist Dr. Stanley Greenspan and child psychologist Dr. Serena Wieder, includes "Regulatory Sensory Processing Disorder" in its *Diagnostic Manual for Infancy and Early Childhood* (ICDL, 2005).

SPD was considered for classification as an independent diagnostic entity by the American Psychiatric Association for the fifth edition of the *Diagnostic and Statistical Manual of Mental Disorders* (*DSM–5*). There was quite a lot of controversy over some of the *DSM–5* revisions, including childhood bipolar disorder and, perhaps most notoriously, the consolidation of autism spectrum diagnoses. SPD did not make it into the final recommendations for the revised edition as an independent diagnostic category.

In 2012, the American Academy of Pediatrics published a report on sensory integration therapy in *Pediatrics* acknowledging the potential benefit of sensory interventions for some children. The academy pointed out that because there is no universally accepted framework for diagnosis, SPD should generally not be diagnosed, noting that it is still unclear whether it can exist as a stand-alone disorder rather than a characteristic of other developmental and behavioral disorders. The academy also stated that occupational therapy services with the use of sensory-based therapies may be acceptable as one of the components of a comprehensive treatment plan.

One of the most positive outcomes of this report is that now all professionals who care for kids and teens—including pediatricians and mental health professionals—know to be on the look-out for sensory processing challenges.

Part II

Using the Best Clinical Strategies

CHAPTER 4

Gaining Insight and Developing a Therapeutic Program

Mental health clinicians can play an essential role in recognizing sensory processing challenges in their clients. A school psychologist may be the first to recognize that sensory processing problems may be causing or contributing to difficulty functioning in the school environment. In the clinic, the psychotherapist may recognize that a client with atypical eating may have underlying sensory defensiveness to food textures and smells. During a crisis, a child with significant mental health issues may arrive at the pediatric psych emergency room and be calmed and reorganized significantly using sensory modulation approaches.

This is why it is so important to be educated about sensory processing issues and to work hand in hand with OTs who have specialized training in sensory modulation, sensorimotor, and sensory discrimination evaluation and intervention. While domains of practice do not always have distinct boundaries—especially when working with children—the best practice for mental health clinicians is to be trained and supervised by an OT colleague when implementing any sensory processing approaches (Champagne & Koomar, 2011). That said, this chapter will walk you through basic treatment considerations and strategies so you'll have a better understanding of what the interventions look like and how they work.

Helping kids and teens with SPD requires a multipronged approach in order to:

1. Protect the child from pain and trauma
2. Assess and increase sensory processing skills
3. Build self-awareness, self-advocacy, and coping skills
4. Educate families, schools, and others

PROTECT THE CHILD FROM PAIN AND TRAUMA

First and foremost, the child must be protected physically and emotionally from pain and trauma. It is essential to make sure that the child does not have any undiagnosed medical issues that may be causing the behavior in question. The colicky baby or biting, fighting child may have an underlying gastrointestinal or dental issue that is making him miserable. A child with special needs and limited ability to communicate what is going on may be banging her head against the bars of her crib because her teeth hurt so much. A more verbal child may be able to communicate that she hurts but be unable to identify where it hurts.

If the child is hurting, every step should be taken to protect that child from pain. For example, when certain sounds are excruciatingly painful, the cause of the pain should be determined (whether it is the sound itself, the sensitivity, an ear infection, etc.), and the child should be protected by being taken away from the sound source or by using ear protection such as noise-reducing headphones. Note that ear protection should not be worn all day. Rather, it should be reserved for times of greatest need to avoid habituation and recalibration of the sensitivity.

There are many less dramatic examples well-intentioned people may not even recognize. Being forced into a disciplinary quiet room at school or another institutional setting because of out-of-bounds behavior is an extreme example of how kids with special needs may be further traumatized. For example, being forced to sit on a hard school chair under fluorescent lights that flicker and hurt the eyes and ears and cause headaches while demanding one make eye contact or perform a certain action can be experienced as anything from unpleasant to hellish. Being placed in a room with soft, diffused incandescent lighting at eye level on a comfortable chair may turn an awful time that triggers some terrible fight-or-flight reactions into a positive learning experience. If a child wanders alone along the shady perimeter of the playground to get as far away as possible from the glare of the sun and chaos of classmates playing dodgeball, give that child some noise-reducing headphones, sunglasses or a cap, and an alternative fun small-group movement activity to do, and you've got a much happier, engaged child.

Create Safe Havens

For children, teens, and adults who are in an overwhelmed, agitated, or even psychotic state, a nurturing sensory retreat is the first line of defense, both in terms of avoiding sensory overload and unwanted behaviors and in terms of recovering from an agitated state. Safe havens take many forms: In a hospital or outpatient clinic it may be a specific sensory room or comfort room, while in a school or at home it may be something along the lines of a relaxation station or just a cozy nook. Whatever it is called, and whether it is a separate room or just a little corner, a safe haven should never be used as a punishment or time-out space, but rather as a strategy for managing arousal level. If the child is overaroused, materials that are calming for that individual should be provided. If the child is having a problem due to low stimulation, more alerting, stimulating materials should be provided.

At Home

Kids and teens often figure out their own safe havens, typically a site in which they can take control of the sensory variables. The classic teenage "chill spot" is a laundry-strewn bedroom, with walls covered with posters and loud music blasting. A younger child may love hanging out with a picture book and a stuffed toy curled up in a soft blanket with a pillow inside a tent in her room. Another may adore a squish box in the form of a large cardboard box or laundry basket filled with pillows or even hanging out in a dark closet with a hand fidget (an object that the child manipulates for self-soothing) where

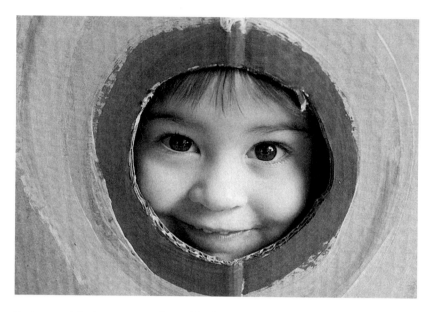

Perla, a spirited sensory seeker with dyspraxia who gets easily overwhelmed, unwinding in one of her favorite comfy spots. *Photo courtesy of Molly Kiely*

she can escape noise and light. For a sensory-seeking child, a safe haven may be a fun zone where he can jump on a trampoline, throw toys around the room, and engage in roughhousing play.

In the Therapy Room

Whether your office is in a small room in a school, a suite of offices, a hospital, or elsewhere, it may deserve some sensory improvements. Whenever possible, turn off overhead fluorescent lighting and use incandescent, warm white LED, or full-spectrum lights on a dimmer. Eliminate or minimize annoying noise from other rooms, heaters, air conditioners, and electrical devices by removing them if possible or by masking them with white or pink noise. White noise, easily obtained through a white noise machine or CD, is created by combining sounds at different frequencies. Pink noise is a consistent frequency of steady, rhythmic sounds such as rain falling or waves breaking. Pink noise slows down and regulates brain waves, creating a relaxed and more restful state. You can add pink noise by playing a pink noise CD or adding a water feature in your office. Provide comfortable seating, ideally offering options such as a plush armchair, rocking chair, bean bag chair, or even a ball chair to meet your client's preferences. Don't forget oral comforts such as water and possibly chewing gum or hard candies if appropriate. Hand fidgets such as squeeze balls should also be available. Of course, do not insist on eye contact and recognize that some clients will be more comfortable facing away from you.

At School

A sensitive child may need to escape to a safe spot at school in order to avoid becoming overloaded. In a classroom, the student might hide in a cubby or under a desk, refusing to come out until she is ready. Creating a safe haven is fairly easy for a young child who can go over to a dimly lit corner of the room, cuddle up on a bean bag chair, put on headphones for noise reduction or to listen to calming music, and look at a picture book while holding a hand fidget. The sensory-seeking student may need an opportunity to engage in organizing activities. Sensory smart classrooms incorporate the sensory tools and movement opportunities described in Chapter 7, depending on students' needs and resources available.

In Mental Health Facilities

Seclusion and restraint protocols are highly stressful for the client in acute distress. The current mandates for reduced restraint and seclusion across mental health care settings recognize this, and sensory rooms show great promise in avoiding further pain and trauma. Nearly 90 percent of adult clients reported decreased distress after the use of a trauma-informed sensory room in a psychiatric inpatient setting (Champagne & Stromberg, 2004; for more on sensory modulation approaches in mental health facilities, see Massachusetts Department of Mental Health, 2007). Most likely, virtually all pediatric clients would find a sensory rooms helpful.

Occupational therapist Dr. Tina Champagne has long championed the use of sensory modulation approaches in mental health facilities, including the use of sensory rooms, consulting with facilities and examining their effectiveness (Champagne, 2006). She noted, "Sensory rooms and spaces are created and used to help people of all ages to

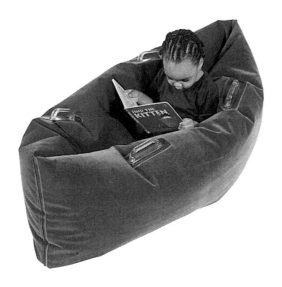

The inflatable Pea Pod Student Calming Station, available in several sizes, helps kids obtain soothing deep pressure. *Photo courtesy of School Specialty*

learn how to change the way they feel, in order to meet their individual needs and goals. These spaces are not to be used for punishment purposes such as time out spaces or for violent and traumatizing procedures such as seclusion or restraint. Rather these can be used to relax, self-nurture, distract, decrease or increase stimulation, and as a healing retreat" (Champagne, personal communication, February 8, 2013).

Of course, children need to learn to function in "the real world," but pain and trauma can make normal function unnecessarily difficult if not totally impossible. Providing a safe haven for the child with significant sensory processing challenges is an essential first step.

Increase Self-Awareness and Self-Advocacy

One of the most important things a parent can do when raising a child is to teach self-soothing. A new mom or dad sings a gentle lullaby or rocks the newborn to help him calm and drift off to sleep. The

infant may use the sucking input of the pacifier to feel secure and satisfied. A parent embraces a toddler when she is upset, reassuring her
that everything will be okay. Soon the young child learns to use self-
talk to work through feelings and problems and to use sensory input
such as listening to favorite songs and dancing, looking at beloved
picture books in a quiet spot, or rubbing a comfort object such as a
soft blanket or toy in order to feel good throughout the day.

As we mature, we continue to use sensory strategies to self-regulate. You may listen to certain music to stay focused while driving or
relaxed while riding mass transit. You may go to the gym before work
to pep up or at the end of the day to wind down. Perhaps you chew
gum, sip water, and take breaks during long, dull meetings.

Of course, if you have always experienced the world in a certain
way, it's hard to imagine that other people experience things differently. Take the child with vision issues who is surprised to learn that
letters actually have clean, stable edges when she finally puts on a
pair of prescription eyeglasses.

Kids with sensory processing problems usually do not have the
self-awareness or autonomy to take the steps they need to keep
themselves on an even keel. It's not as if a student can simply walk
out of class because she's bored and antsy and thinks a 10-minute
jog around the building would help her feel much better. A child may
not even recognize that he has low energy or is hyped up in the first
place, not to mention knowing acceptable options for dealing with
this. Instead, he'll act out in ways that may be unacceptable such as
falling asleep, clowning around, and being disruptive.

The clinician may need to teach the client to be more self-obser-
vant and to catch herself before she has a problem. This requires self-
knowledge and an understanding of the sensory environment, most
notably the particular factors that can be problematic. "When I get
overstimulated I just want to *get out*. I can't focus on anything except
keeping myself together and regaining control of my body. I'm learning to self-regulate instead of dropping on to the floor and hitting
myself and screaming" (seventh grader).

Lynn Soraya (2013), an adult with Asperger's syndrome, writes in her *Psychology Today* blog about sitting at her computer at the end of the day and being overcome by "billowing rage," wanting to scream and throw her computer for no obvious reason. She describes taking mental time out, breathing, and analyzing what caused the episode, realizing it was the consequence of an unpleasant sensory experience earlier that day at a crowded library book sale. "Whenever I thought I'd accommodated to the uncomfortably loud, but steady, strong morass of sound, someone's voice would leap out of the crowd louder than the rest, as if they'd suddenly appeared immediately next to my ear, or someone had cranked the volume on a stereo to maximum without warning," she writes. "A few moments of that, and I began to feel like I'd been whipped, repeatedly." She eventually made her way through the throngs of people and, once sufficiently calm, drove home and curled up on the couch with a blanket. Hours later, suddenly becoming angry at the computer, she realized, "this is what comes of spending most of my life suppressing my differences instead of trying to understand them. Sensory overload is an assault. . . . Recovering from an assault takes more than just removing yourself from the situation. It has emotional after-effects, too. Ones that can affect not only you, but those around you."

Developing such self-awareness and insight takes maturity and, often, some extra help. Rather than aiming to teach clients to suppress sensory differences, clinicians can help kids, teens, and adults learn to recognize internal and environmental experiences that are potential irritants, predict situations that will be problematic, and use the best strategies to overcome them.

Troublesome sensations can be explored through use of a simple questionnaire for a teenager or young adult with a lot of insight into his own sensory preferences and intolerances. However, for many teens and certainly younger children, it will take clinical observations in the field as well as direct experimentation in the clinic such as touching an assortment of objects and fabrics, trying different kinds of movement such as rocking in a chair and bouncing on a therapy ball, sniffing different essential oils, and so on.

ASSESS AND INCREASE SENSORY SKILLS

Once the child or teen is no longer in pain, the starting place is, quite logically, getting a clearer picture of sensory difficulties and their impact on the life of the child and family. A good way to start is with the Sensory Screening Tool for home and school provided in Chapter 2. Remember that screening is just that: a quick look at whether sensory issues might be a factor and whether a comprehensive sensory processing evaluation is warranted. In addition to the screening tools in this book, there are commercially available questionnaires. Two of the most widely used sensory questionnaires are:

- Sensory Profile (Dunn, 1999). This self-administered questionnaire contains 125 questions for parents and caregivers about sensory processing skills, reactions, and behaviors. It is standardized for children from age 3 to age 10 years, 11 months with mild to moderate variations in physical and intellectual abilities, including autism spectrum disorders. There is also the Infant/Toddler Sensory Profile (Dunn, 2002), Adolescent/Adult Sensory Profile (Brown & Dunn, 2002), and Sensory Profile School Companion for classroom teachers (Dunn, 2006). All Sensory Profile tests are discriminant, determining whether a child has sensory reactions and behaviors that differ from those of the average child. As such, the Sensory Profile cannot be used to measure progress over time.

- Sensory Processing Measure (Parham & Ecker; Kuhaneck, Henry, & Glennon, 2007). There are three parts to this standardized questionnaire for parents and teachers that assesses sensory processing, praxis and motor planning, and social participation in children ages 5–12: a home form, a main classroom form, and a school environments form (for the bus, art, music, physical education, playground or recess, and the cafeteria). Any combination of forms may be administered: just the home part, just the classroom part, just a few school environments, or all. There is a preschool version for children ages 2–5. The Sensory Processing Measure is standardized for children with a wider range of physical and intellectual abilities than the Sensory Profile, including lower-functioning children with autism. Because this test focuses on performance rather than discrimination between average and atypical sensory skills, it may be repeated at intervals to measure progress over time.

Data collection through questionnaires alone is just the beginning. Any questionnaires should, of course, be supplemented by discussion as well as observation in natural settings such as the home and school environment, discussions with clients and their caregivers, and coordinated with findings from other disciplines. As sensory processing skills form the basis of all other developmental skills—such as fine motor, gross motor, and visual perceptual skills—it is best to refer to an OT for a specialized evaluation. Collaborating with other professionals is addressed more fully in Chapter 5.

Learning About Sensory Vulnerabilities

All too often, children, teens, or even adults with sensory issues will become annoyed, frustrated, and upset with a person or situation due to sensory disturbances they can't identify and do not know how to deal with. The child with autism who bangs her head each afternoon may be reacting to what she ate for lunch, the smell of her aide's breath after she eats and then brushes her teeth, being overstimulated by recess, the afternoon's challenging math activity, anticipation of a dreaded afterschool activity, or a combination of all of those things.

You might teach your clients about the concept of a sensory SNAFU (SNAFU stands for Situation Normal, All Fouled Up). Sensory SNA-FUs can completely undermine the person with sensory issues. It may be an entirely "normal" situation, but it's all fouled up for that person due to sensory processing issues. Some clients may be able to pinpoint precisely what sensory experiences bug them. Others require exploration and perhaps parents, teachers, and other caregivers to parse out sensory input that is troublesome. As your sensitive client matures and learns what sets her off, she can increasingly articulate what bothers her and learn to self-advocate.

SENSORY CHALLENGE QUESTIONNAIRE

The Sensory Challenge Questionnaire can be completed by a high-functioning older child, teen, or young adult in identifying personal SNAFUs or as an interview guideline to assist you in exploring what is happening in your client's sensory world. Please feel free to duplicate the Sensory Challenge Questionnaire in this book or you can download it from sensoryprocessingchallenges.com.

Tactile

What touch experiences are challenging for you?

Please consider activities such as wearing clothing and shoes, brushing teeth, washing face and hair, using lotion, being touched by others, getting hands messy, food textures, temperature and pain experiences, and so on.

_____

_____

_____

_____

_____

_____

What touch experiences do you enjoy?

_____

_____

_____

_____

_____

_____

Auditory

What sound experiences are challenging for you?

Please consider activities such as listening to people talking in both quiet and noisy situations, any annoying sounds, reactions to loud or unexpected noises, musical styles or musical instruments, ability to follow verbal directions, and so on.

_____

_____

_____

_____

_____

What sound experiences do you enjoy?

_____

_____

_____

_____

_____

Visual

What visual experiences are challenging for you?

Please consider visual demands such as reading, locating items in a crowded visual field, being in busy environments such as shopping malls, types of lighting (fluorescent, incandescent, downcast lights, sunshine, darkness, etc.), patterns, colors, contrasts, objects in your peripheral vision, watching moving objects, and so on.

_____

_____

_____

_____

_____

_____

What visual experiences do you enjoy?

_____

_____

_____

_____

_____

Gustatory (Taste) and Food

What taste experiences are challenging for you?

Please consider tastes (sweet, salty, sour, bitter, and savory) as well as particular foods that you strongly dislike in terms of flavor, temperature, or texture (chewy, crunchy, dry and crumbly, slippery, mixed textures), and so on.

_____

_____

_____

_____

_____

_____

What flavors and foods do you enjoy?

_____

_____

_____

_____

_____

Olfactory (Smell)

What smell experiences are challenging for you?

Please consider factors such as perfumes, body lotions, clean-ing products, food aromas, garbage smells, nature scents, inanimate objects that have a particular smell, and so on.

_____

_____

_____

_____

_____

What smell experiences do you enjoy?

_____

_____

_____

_____

_____

_____

Vestibular (Movement)

What movement experiences are challenging for you?

Please consider activities such as walking, running, climbing stairs, having your head upside down, spinning, swinging, sitting still, rocking, riding in a car, airplane or other mode of transportation, engaging in sports, and so on.

_____

_____

_____

_____

_____

_____

_____

What movement experiences do you enjoy?

_____

_____

_____

_____

_____

_____

_____

Proprioception (Body Awareness)

What proprioceptive experiences are challenging for you?

Please consider times when you feel uncoordinated, awkward, weaker than others, or "lost in space," whether you look closely at what you are doing, or whether it is hard for you to learn new activities like tying your shoelaces, riding a bike, skating, and so on.

_____

_____

_____

_____

_____

_____

What proprioceptive experiences do you enjoy?

_____

_____

_____

_____

_____

More Formal Curricula

To supplement your one-to-one clinical practice, there are a variety of structured programs you might consider using with individual clients and groups to help build insights into sensory modulation and self-regulation vulnerabilities, including these:

• The Zones of Regulation (Kuypers, 2011) is a cognitive-behavioral curriculum designed by an OT to teach self-regulation and emotional control, categorizing states of alertness and emotion using colored zones comparable to traffic signals. For example, the Green Zone is used for the regulated, calm, controlled state needed for schoolwork and socializing, while the Red Zone is used for extremely heightened states of alertness or very intense feelings such as rage or terror. The curriculum is designed to help students recognize when they are in each zone and what they can do to help themselves move to a different zone (for more information, visit zonesofregulation.com).

- The Sensory Modulation Program (Champagne, 2011) helps to train interdisciplinary staff to use sensory modulation approaches. It was initially created for use with adolescents and adults in mental health facilities such as acute inpatient psychiatric units, but has been modified for use with a variety of populations and settings (e.g., educational, residential, forensic). Components include therapeutic use of self, sensory-based assessments, sensorimotor activities, sensory-based modalities, programming, and environmental modifications (for more information, visit ot-innovations.com).

- The SMART Model: Sensory Motor Arousal Regulation Treatment (Warner, Cook, Westcott, & Koomar, 2011) was created by psychotherapists and an OT to support arousal regulation in children and teens with trauma symptoms and diagnoses in clinics, residential treatment sites, and schools. The SMART model provides a framework for integrating sensory processing approaches with psychotherapeutic approaches such as trauma and attachment frames of reference as well as body-oriented therapies such as sensorimotor psychotherapy (for more information, visit traumacenter.org/clients/SMART.php).

- The Integrated Self-Advocacy ISA Curriculum (Paradiz, 2009) is designed to help people with disabilities such as autism to self-advocate. A key part of this curriculum is the ISA Sensory Scan, designed to help users learn to scan a particular room or environment for sensory challenges, rate the level of the challenge, then develop a sensory advocacy plan to address specific needs or prepare requests for accommodations. ISA offers online courses, including professional certification (for more information visit autismselfadvocacy.com).

- The Alert Program (Williams & Shellenberger, 1996) with its companion book *How Does Your Engine Run?* helps parents, teachers, and therapists to teach self-regulation awareness and ways to improve or maintain states of alertness. The program was initially created for children ages 8–12 with attention and learning difficulties using the concrete analogy that the body is like a car engine that sometimes runs on high, sometimes on low, and sometimes just right. The Alert Program has been adapted for ages preschool through adult and for a variety of disabilities (for more information, visit alertprogram.com).

SENSORY TOOLS AND ACTIVITIES TO CONSIDER

Helping clients become aware of their sensory processing challenges is the cornerstone of any therapeutic program. Once clients have some insight, they can begin to proactively seek out sensory solutions that will help them feel better.

People with serious sensory issues, such as the sensory scrambling seen in autism, may not be able to pinpoint exactly what it is in the environment that is causing them such distress. Jeremy Sicile-Kira, a 24-year-old autism advocate and coauthor of *A Full Life With Autism: From Learning to Forming Relationships to Achieving Independence*, shares, "One day I went to the store for flowers for a school project. The store had very bright fluorescent lights that I could not see. I could not feel my body. I had to leave right away. I was afraid I would wet my pants as this happened to me before in a similarly lit store" (Sicile-Kira, personal communication, February 6, 2013). You'll read more about Jeremy in Chapter 8.

Chloe Rothschild is a 21-year-old autism advocate who blogs for Special-ism and her own blog, Oh, the Places I'll Go: My Life With Autism blog. In personal correspondence she writes:

> I have sound sensitivity, though not as intense as it used to be. Unexpected loud noises tend to startle me, like when I was at the mall and the fire alarm went off. I started to scream because it was loud and I was not expecting the fire alarm to go off at the mall. If the fire alarm goes off at school, it is okay because I know fire drills happen at school. When I was younger attending school assemblies was somewhat challenging for me because the loud noises, especially the noise of the band playing, made me anxious and uncomfortable. It was just too loud. I have noise canceling headphones that I use if noises are bothering me. I also have headphones that I

use to listen to music that I find to be very calming. I usually listen to the same song over and over.

I need movement—frequently and lots of it. The movement helps me focus and to calm my body when I am feeling overwhelmed, anxious, or uncomfortable. I like to sit in office chairs with wheels because I enjoy moving in them. I also enjoy swinging, sitting in a rocking chair, pacing and walking. Sometimes when I feel dysregulated I get this yucky feeling in my body: I feel hot, my head hurts, and my stomach feels sick. The good news is that this feeling does not tend to last that long, and there are things that I've learned to do in order to help myself feel regulated again. (Rothschild, personal communication, January 30, 2013)

A key role you can take with clients who have sensory issues is to help them to recognize which sensory strategies will help them attain and maintain that well-regulated, calm yet alert state we all strive for when out and about in the world. The checklist of sensory modulation tools and activities in the pages ahead will give you some ideas to explore, though you will need to tailor suggestions to the needs and resources of each client.

Remember that you are helping the person to self-modulate arousal level and that these activities and tools in themselves do not build sensory processing skills. For that, you will need to work with an OT who can assess skill deficits and recommend interventions that aim to specifically rewire the central nervous system. Nevertheless, using sensory strategies and modulation tools frequently enables a person to adjust to different levels of sensory stimulation and empowers the individual to take charge of his sensory experiences.

In Chapters 6 and 7, you will learn sensory strategies for handling real-life challenges in both the home and school setting, including ways to modify tasks and the environment. Taken together, these sensory modulation tools and activities plus environmental and task modifications make up a sensory program that many OTs refer to as a "sensory diet" (see Chapter 5).

In the clinic, you can explore some sensory modulation tools and activities the clients may use in various contexts to help their bodies to feel better and to stay better self-regulated, helping them feel empowered to take how they feel into their own hands. As you explore sensory modulation tools, be sure to consider whether your goal is to identify calming or alerting input. What any one person will find calming or alerting is certainly idiosyncratic. You may become agitated when you hear hip-hop music while your client finds it helps her focus. You may be enthralled with the smell of scented candles while your client finds them nauseating.

Also consider age appropriateness. For example, having a teenager use Play-Doh may be perceived as infantilizing by the client, peers, or caregivers. You may want to give this client Sculpey craft clay or Crazy Aaron's Thinking Putty instead. Or you can put the Play-Doh in a container with no label so the client doesn't associate it with small children. All of these items should be referred to as "tools" and not "toys" to promote acceptance in older children as well as to increase school staff's willingness to incorporate such items into daily classroom routines. Children may not be allowed to bring toys into class, but "sensory tools" are more readily accepted.

Sensory exploration can be fun and exciting, a journey you and clients can take together one on one or in a group. Most of the supplies and equipment mentioned are readily available and reasonably priced. There are some general usage and selection principles that you can use as a guide, based on the following:

- Rhythmicity: Does the input follow a steady pattern or is it erratic? Which is best for the client in which situations? For example, if a child is overstimulated, it may help to have him sit in a rocking chair and rhythmically rock back and forth until he is calm. In a state of low arousal, your client may benefit from rocking back and forth less predictably, for example, 10 times then stopping, 2 times then stopping, 5 times then stopping, using this erratic vestibular input to activate his nervous system rather than to calm it down.

- Familiarity versus novelty: How much does this client crave familiarity and repetition—and does this lead to a state of calm or tuned-out self-absorption? How much novelty is required to maintain interest without overstimulation?

- Intensity: How intense is the input? Does the intensity match the person's needs or overwhelm him?
- Frequency: How often does the person need this input in order for it to be effective? Every hour? Once a day? Once a week?
- Duration: How long should the input be used?

Again, consultation with an OT is strongly recommended when considering sensory exploration tools for a client.

As you explore sensory experiences that are challenging for your client, you can begin introducing tools and techniques that might help, including strategies for modifying environments and activities that you'll find in the following chapters, as well as sensory tools the person may be able to use to help himself feel and function better. The following are some possibilities.

Tactile

- Use hand fidgets including smooth and textured items such as squeeze balls, hand exercisers like the Eggsercizer or Pediatools monkey, worry stones, stuffed toys, or fabrics such as corduroy and velvet.
- Use clay: Play-Doh, Aroma Dough or Wonder Dough for gluten-free kids, Eco Kids Eco-Dough for chemically sensitive kids, Silly Putty, Gak, Floam, Model Magic, Sculpey, Kinetic Sand, strength-graded Putty Elements, Crazy Aaron's Thinking Putty for older kids and teens, Theraputty, modeling clay, and others.
- Water: Take a warm or cool shower or bath, swim, snorkel, scuba dive, or use a water table.
- Firm massage with or without lotion.
- Use a backscratcher, washcloth, loofah, or net scrubber in the shower.
- Deep-pressure brushing and joint compressions (consult with an OT for training).
- Deep pressure: bear hugs; swaddle or roll up like a burrito in a blanket or thin exercise mat with head out; log rolling; jumping on a crash pad; "sandwich" between pillows or sofa cushions; use a Steamroller Squeeze machine; roll over a therapy ball.

• Arts and crafts such as drawing with markers, crayons, colored pencils, painting, glitter glue, modeling clay, crochet, knitting, sewing.

• Messy play with foaming soap, shaving cream, pudding, mud, whipped cream.

• Cooking, using hands or tools to mix, break up ingredients, and so on.

• Sandbox or sensory bin with dry rice and beans or other materials.

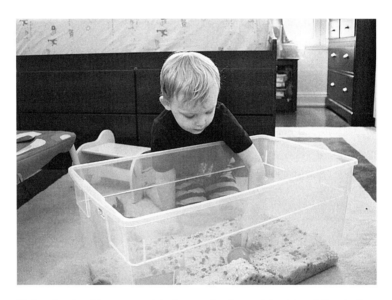

Richard using his sensory bin for tactile desensitization while playing. Sensory bins can be customized with materials ranging from mixed textures like uncooked rice and beans to shaving cream. *Photo courtesy of the author*

• Gardening, especially a sensory garden with fragrant, hardy plants you can touch.

• Vibration: vibrating chairs at nail salon or for use at home and school from stores like Brookstone; sit on a washing machine; vibrating massagers (Z-Vibe, Jigglers, animal massagers); vibrating pens (e.g., Squiggle Wiggle Writer, Tran-Quille); vibrating toys (e.g., Bumble Ball); vibrating pillows (e.g., Senseez, Vibrating Love Bug); vibrating hairbrush and toothbrush; Vibramat under furniture; Tender Vibes mattress.

Using Weight and Compression

Weight

Many children, teens, and adults respond positively to feeling weight on their skin, muscles, joints, and connective tissue by sleeping under a heavy blanket, wearing a full backpack, lifting weights, and so on. Weighted wearables increase sensory cues to the body using the downward force of gravity to create input and come in a variety of forms including weighted blankets, lap pads, shoulder wraps, vests, hoodies, hats, and stuffed toys. Typical weight recommendations are 5–10 percent of body weight (e.g., 50 lbs: 2–5 lbs weight), but an OT or physical therapist may experiment with somewhat lighter or heavier weight. Typical wearing times are 20 minutes on, 20 minutes off in order to prevent the person from becoming habituated to the input.

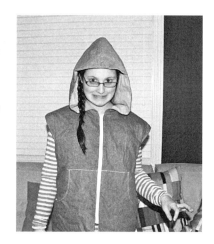

Chloe Rothschild wearing her weighted hoodie from Sensory Critters. *Photo courtesy of Susan Dolin Rothschild*

Some people will benefit from a longer wearing time. People productively engaged in an activity should not be interrupted in order to remove the weighted item.

Weighted blankets are obviously worn differently than a weighted vest and are not necessarily subject to the same usage recommendations. Tina Champagne has pioneered studies on the safety and efficacy of using weighted blankets to reduce anxiety with adult mental health populations, developing her Weighted Blanket Competency-Based Training Program (Champagne, 2011). More research needs to be conducted with younger populations regarding weight and duration of use for short-term calming input as well as to promote more restful sleep.

Compression

Other people benefit from the sensation of compression from confirming, snug clothing such as Lycra sportswear and control-top tights. Compression garments give tactile and deep pressure input that, when properly applied, supports muscle tone, postural control, and body awareness. Because of the four-way dynamic stretch, compression garments may be worn all day.

Weighted and compression items may be homemade or easily found in many OT/PT catalogs and online. For weighted items, see weightedwearables.com, miraclebelt.com, sensacalm.com, sommerfly.com, sensorycritters.com, stitchesbyAnne.info, cozycalm.com, weightedblanket.net, and many others. For compression garments, see underarmour.com, SPIOworks.com, squeasewear.com,velvasoft.com, and others.

- Pet a dog, cat, or other animal.
- Play a musical instrument such as strumming a guitar.
- Use a compression garment or weighted vest, blanket, lap pad, or other weighted item.
- For children who are extremely heat-sensitive, consider a cooling vest such as the StaCool child vest (stacoolvest.com).

Auditory

- Enjoy a quiet space.
- Listen to the sounds of nature including animals, water, and wind while playing, working, or falling asleep.
- Play music that is calming or music that is alerting. Consider classical or pop music, pure instrumental or singing, nature recordings, and slow steady beats or faster beats.
- Bang on pots and pans (young children) or drums.
- Whisper, sing, or hum.
- Blow a whistle or kazoo.
- Use a white noise machine or white or pink noise CD.
- Use a metronome to provide a steady beat during any activity.

Vision

- Take a break in soft ambient lighting.
- Relax eyes strained by close-up work (writing, computers, reading) by gazing into the distance approximately every 20 minutes.
- Look at a relaxing photograph, DVD, or picture book (popular themes include animals, landscapes, great paintings).
- Look at a fish tank, mobiles, lava lamps, bubble lamps.
- Wear tinted lenses indoors to cut glare.
- Wear optical-quality sunglasses and/or wide brim hats outdoors.
- Use colored overlays on printed material (see irlen.com and autismtoday.com/colored-reading-overlays.php).

Dealing With Sound Sensitivity

Step 1: Protect. Safeguard ultrasensitive ears by using earplugs, noise-canceling head-phones, or sound-reducing earmuffs. You'll find these at your local drugstore, music sup-plier, or hardware store. An excellent online resource is earplugstore.com, which offers a wide variety of high-quality sound-protecting earmuffs for babies, children, adults, and even dogs. Make sure the person does not wear ear protection all day because the brain and auditory system will get used to the dampened sound. Save them for specific situations that are especially challenging.

Step 2: Desensitize. Kids with sensory issues may overcome some of their overreactivity through repeated exposure. It may help to record the offending sound and listen to it together in a different context in which the child can control the volume and turn it on and off. You can also listen to selections from Sound-Eaze and School-Eaze CDs (route2great-ness.com), which pair many of the sounds children are most afraid of such as the vacuum cleaner, blender, toilet flushing, fire alarm, and thunder with pleasant, rhythmic songs to help the child predict and tolerate distressing sounds.

Step 3: Increase skills. Work with an OT, speech language pathologist, or audiologist who has expertise in building sensory tolerance and processing skills. Sound-based therapy programs such as Therapeutic Listening, Integrated Listening Systems (iLs), Solisten, and others are designed to strengthen and integrate the person's auditory system with other sensory and motor systems. Software programs such as Earobics and Fast ForWord help build auditory processing skills. Meanwhile, the child may benefit from an FM Unit in the classroom to bring the teacher's voice to the foreground, empowering the student to hear her voice more strongly than classmates or ambient noise.

Step 4: Build advocacy. Teach clients and families to advocate for themselves in a polite but assertive manner. For example, a student can learn to ask the teacher to repeat an instruction and a teenager at a restaurant can politely ask the waiter or hostess to lower the music if he is unable to hear his friends.

Children who are overwhelmed by the volume of movies might especially enjoy AMC's Sensory Friendly Films series in which first-run films are shown at lower volume with raised house lights, snacks from home are welcome, and kids can move and talk as needed (see AMCtheatres.com/programs/sensory-friendly-films).

Smell, Taste, and Oral Comforts

- Explore high-quality pure essential oils such as vanilla, rose, and sweet orange (which tend to be calming) and lemon, peppermint, and eucalyptus (which tend to be invigorating).
- Smell flowers, spices, and herbs.
- Explore tastes: sweet, salty, sour, spicy, bitter.
- Eat frozen, cool, or warm foods.

Safe Computer Use

To reduce the risk of visual strain as well as neck, shoulder, wrist, and back pain while working on a computer, users should do the following:

- Use an ergonomic, adjustable task chair with lumbar support so that ankles, hips, knees, and elbows are bent at roughly 90 degrees.
- The screen should be at eye level so that the user doesn't have to bend to see.
- Adjust screen brightness so that it is roughly equivalent to room brightness.
- Position the computer monitor so that windows are to the side rather than in front or back.
- Reduce lighting in the room by closing shades and dimming lights.
- Look at a distant object outside or down the hallway to relax focused eye muscles every 20 minutes.
- Blink eyes 10 times to rewet them every 20 minutes.
- Get up and move around once an hour.

- Explore textures: crunchy, creamy, chewy, lumpy, and so on.
- Drink water.
- Chew gum (see Chapter 7).
- Drink a carbonated beverage or slushie.
- Blow: for example, bubbles, Blo Pens, whistles.
- Suck on a mint, lollipop, or hard candy.
- Suck thick liquid through a straw.
- Use an age-appropriate "chewy" you'll find in OT and speech therapy catalogs such as a Chewy Tube, Ark Grabber, KidCompanions Chewelry, ChewEase Pencil Topper, Teething Bling, Dr. Bloom's Chewable Jewels, Chew Stixx (chewstixx.com), Chewelry, or terry cloth wristbands.

Movement and Body Awareness

- Rocking (parent's arms, hobby horse, glider, or rocking chair).
- Walking, marching, and running.
- Wheelbarrow walking.
- Jump on trampoline, do jumping jacks.
- Use swings and slides.
- Climb stairs.

> **Words of Caution**
>
> Never, ever force sensory stimulation on a child, teen, or adult. Watch out for signs of physi-
> ological overload such as increased distractibility, disorientation, nausea, skin reddening or
> paleness, breathing changes, and unexpected behaviors.

- Use Sit 'n Spin, Dizzy Disc Jr., or other spinning toy.
- Use a hop ball or Rockin' Rody.
- Bounce on a therapy ball.
- Ride a tricycle, bicycle, scooter, or skateboard.
- Sports and gymnastics.
- Yoga and Pilates.
- Swimming.
- Dancing.
- Mindfulness meditation.
- Horseback riding.
- Lift weights, do push-ups, pull-ups, and sit-ups.
- Ice skating, sledding, skiing.
- Cleaning, gardening, laundry.

Managing Stims

Self-stimulatory behaviors such as hand flapping, rocking, and staring at spinning objects are repetitive actions most often associated
with autism, but are seen in a variety of diagnoses. As Temple Grandin (2011) wisely points out, not all repetitive behaviors are stims, so
it is important to distinguish the source behind the behavior:

- Stimming behaviors. These behaviors self-soothe a child and
  help him regain emotional balance. Unfortunately, if children are
  allowed to stim all day, no learning will take place because the
  child's brain is shut off from the outside world.
- Involuntary movements. These movements can resemble stims
  but may be caused by either Tourette's syndrome (TS) or tardive
  dyskinesia, a side effect of antipsychotic drugs such as Risperdal

(risperidone), Seroquel (quetiapine), or Abilify (aripiprazole). The nerve damage—sometimes permanent—from these drugs causes the repetitive behaviors.

• Meltdown due to sensory overload. When this happens, the child is often having an outburst while exhibiting repetitive behaviors like kicking or flapping. The best approach is to get the child to a quiet place and let him calm down.

The repetitive behaviors due to TS or tardive dyskinesia or even in the throes of a complete sensory meltdown are more or less involuntary. In contrast, stimming is relatively voluntary, although it may be done unconsciously. Far from nonpurposeful as typically labeled, stims serve several very useful functions, helping a person to:

• Block out overwhelming sensory input (e.g., humming to override too much noise in a room) or painful sensations (e.g., banging head due to toothache) by becoming absorbed in a repetitive action.

• Communicate needs to others when he is upset, hungry, tired, or bored.

• Manage both positive and negative emotions, hand flapping when excited and throwing objects or biting when frustrated or angry.

• Regulate a poorly functioning nervous system by revving it up (e.g., jumping or biting oneself) or calming it down (e.g., rocking or clicking).

• Provide a sense of control and mastery when used to organize the environment (e.g., lining up toys).

• Generate feelings of pleasure or anesthesia since stim behaviors are thought to produce beta endorphins, the body's own painkillers.

Truth is, we all stim to some extent for the very same reasons. You may pinch your own hand when you are getting a shot to block out the pain, tap your fingers on the table or check your e-mail excessively in front of others, which nonverbally (and rudely) indicates you are bored, go for a brisk walk around the block to wake up at midday, line up things on your desk when you are swamped with work, or exercise for that natural runner's high. Like most symptoms, the key is whether the behavior limits and impairs everyday functioning. The child engaged in self-stimulatory behavior for hours each day loses out on essential time for learning, playing, and socializing. The person engaged in endorphin-generating behaviors wants to repeat the activity to maintain those good feelings, so the behavior becomes an addiction. Demanding that the child stop or preventing him from stimming on a particular object by taking it away is usually ineffective because the behavior serves a purpose. Remove the child's car with the wheels he likes to spin, and he'll spin crayons on a table. Punish a child for humming and she'll tap on surfaces. Take away preferred modes of self-soothing and the child may be even less able to stay regulated and further withdraw into herself or act out in a way that alienates and upsets others.

A more effective approach is to analyze what is causing the excessive stimming and to either eliminate the need, distract the child, redirect the behavior, or make it more functional.

Your analysis should examine these considerations:

- Is there an underlying medical cause? This is something to consider, especially when the stim has a sudden onset; for example, a child who suddenly starts swiping at her ears or banging her head out of nowhere may have an ear infection or headache. Sudden onset of grinding teeth may indicate a toothache, jaw pain, or even a stomachache or headache.

- In which circumstances and under what conditions the child stims. Were there too many unexpected changes in routine? Too many abrupt transitions between activities? Is she overwhelmed by the sensory, social, or academic demands of the environment? Does it happen with anyone in particular? In any location in particular?

- What the person gets out of the behavior. Does it help him release pent-up energy? Help him to soothe himself? Is he telling others to back off? That he needs a break? Does it bring attention he craves?

- What sensory system(s) are affected?

  - Tactile, such as rubbing, tapping, scratching, touching, pulling hair, mouthing objects or body parts, head banging?

  - Auditory, such as humming, making odd noises, echolalia, singing, banging, tapping ears, listening to the same song repeatedly, excessive, inappropriate giggling?

- – Visual, such as flicking fingers in front of face, shaking or side-to-side head movements, staring at lights or shiny objects, opening and closing doors and drawers, or spinning objects?

- – Vestibular and proprioceptive, such as rocking, spinning, hanging upside down, jumping, running, pacing, hopping, bouncing?

- – Taste and smell, such as sniffing, licking or biting nonfood objects without eating, smelling people and toys, seeking out strong and even repugnant smells?

Stimming for a moment now and then is not a big deal, but a child who spends a lot of time on self-absorbed stim behavior needs help engaging in activities that will actually help her to develop socially, emotionally, and neurodevelopmentally.

Once you have achieved some understanding of why the child is stimming, then you can make an informed plan regarding what to do about it. Here are some techniques:

- • Attempt to redirect the behavior by giving the child something more appealing to do. If he is jumping, bring out a mini trampoline and count his jumps, or have him sit on a therapy ball and count his bounces, having him stop every so often. If she licks objects, give her an ice pop or lollipop to lick instead. Occupational therapists typically will assess stim behaviors and make them part of a program of activities that meet the underlying sensory needs in a time- and context-appropriate way.

- • Make a connection. If a child is rolling a car back and forth over and over, join the play with another car and teach the child how to scaffold on play themes such as obstructing the way, crashing into it, racing, building a road, and so on. For a child who is intensely self-absorbed in humming, having someone else hum alongside him instead of insisting that he stop may be a welcome surprise. Teach him to hum or sing a song, or to learn to play the song on a xylophone or piano. Dr. Stanley Greenspan's Floortime Approach, with its premise that adults can help children expand their circles of communication by meeting them at their developmental level and building on their strengths, is an evidence-based approach that is well suited to making such connections (see stanleygreenspan.com).

- • Schedule time-limited, location-specific stim time as part of the child's daily routine. For example, she might be given 10 minutes after school to sit at her sensory table and dribble sand through her fingers while rocking in her chair. Use a timer as discussed in Chapter 6.

• Reduce internal and environmental stressors if you believe they are contributing to the stims. Is the room too bright? Is it too noisy? Is the child hungry? Does she need a nap or simply some time to chill out and relax? You'll find many strategies for doing this in Chapters 6 and 7.

EDUCATE OTHERS ABOUT SENSORY ISSUES

One of the most important ways you can help kids, teens, and their families is to educate them—and everyone they interact with—to increase understanding, compassion, and willingness to incorporate sensory strategies. Remember that other family members or friends may be judgmental about how a parent appears to cater to her son's eating likes and dislikes or seems to be less strict about behaviors than she ought to be. The last thing the parent of a child in the midst of a sensory meltdown wants is for others to offer help and well-meaning advice—or worse yet, to hear she's raising a brat or something along the lines of "Give that kid one week in my house and he'd give up that nonsense."

"If a child experiences a sensory meltdown in public, parents should take a few deep breaths, tune out the eye-rolling onlookers who offer unsolicited advice or judgments, and focus on the safety and well-being of the child," suggests Ida Zelaya, president of Sensory Street, Inc., and a certified health and wellness counselor. "You can prepare yourself with a short script about what's going on with your child," Zelaya advises. To make this easier, Zelaya offers a download-able calling card to explain the child's behavior (see appendix). "You never know, the onlookers might be more sensitive the next time they are in the vicinity of a public meltdown," she says (Zelaya, personal communication, February 23, 2013).

Bryan G., the parent of a school-age boy with sensory issues, says, "I don't give a s--t what a stranger thinks. But I might say, 'My child has sensory processing disorder. It is a medical condition that makes it painful for him to take in the sensory input of the world around them. Please be patient and understanding while he takes some time to get accustomed to this environment'" (Bryan G., personal communication, February 25, 2013).

If the onlooker or in-law is particularly rude, a parent might go so far as to add, "My child is also working on improving his social skills such as being polite. That's something you might want to think about for yourself."

Meanwhile, remind clients and families that knowledge is a very powerful thing. Ample resources are available to help educate those who have never heard of sensory processing issues or who say, "Oh, that's the new diagnosis du jour. I don't believe in it." In addition to the book you are now reading, there are many trade books for parents, teachers, and others, including *Raising a Sensory Smart Child: The Definitive Handbook for Helping Your Child With Sensory Processing Issues* (Biel & Peske, 2009; for additional resources, please see the appendix). It may also help to share a simple handout explaining how SPD affects a child, such as the graphic poster "Do You Know Me?" (see Appendix).

Remember, the more others know, the more they'll be willing to help. Often some fairly simple accommodations can make all the difference. You'll find accommodations and modifications for school and home in Chapters 6 and 7. Meanwhile, it's important to educate yourself about the different professionals you may need to collaborate with to make the greatest impact on your client with sensory issues.

CHAPTER 5

Collaborating With Occupational Therapists and Other Professionals

Hillary Rodham Clinton, a longtime advocate for children, wrote that "it takes a village" to enable children to become empowered and resilient adults. This is especially true when helping kids and teens with sensory processing challenges.

The gold standard of treatment for sensory processing issues has always been occupational therapy from a therapist with extensive training and experience in sensory integration theory and practice. Some OTs work alongside psychiatrists, psychologists, social workers, and other clinicians in mental health facilities while many others work in schools, hospitals, and other practice settings.

OTs and mental health clinicians make perfect partners, treating the whole child by addressing the full spectrum of emotional and physical needs. The OT builds sensory processing, neuromuscular, motor, psychosocial, and other developmental skills, enabling the child to better explore his world, while the mental health clinician cultivates the client's self-awareness, coping skills, and ability to self-advocate in positive, prosocial ways.

It may help to think of the OT as taking a more bottom-up approach and the mental health clinician as taking a more top-down approach. In other words, the OT builds the neural pathways between the brain and the body, resulting in a change in how the client feels and thinks, while the mental health clinician builds the psychosocial and emotional skills resulting in a change in how the client feels and thinks. The end goal is identical: to help the client become competent, confident, productive, and as independent as possible in daily life.

WHAT IS OCCUPATIONAL THERAPY?

Occupational therapy is a health care profession that uses functional, purposeful activities to help people engage optimally in meaningful life occupations, which includes taking care of one's body, playing and socializing, attending school, and going to work. OTs work in schools, hospitals, rehabilitation centers, outpatient clinics, private practice, community organizations, and other settings. With training in areas such as psychology and psychiatry, anatomy and physiology, neurology and orthopedics, OTs facilitate development, increase independence, and prevent or minimize disability for people of all ages with emotional, developmental, physical, or social difficulties. Physical therapists (PTs) have a specific focus on neuromuscular and orthopedic issues, discussed later in this chapter.

In addition to evaluating and treating the sensory processing challenges discussed throughout this book, OTs who treat children may address these areas:

- Fine motor skills such as hand grasp and release, managing closures such as buttons and shoelaces, and use of tools like crayons and scissors.
- Gross motor skills such as climbing stairs and using playground equipment.
- Motor planning skills in order to engage in unfamiliar movement patterns.
- Self-help skills such as self-feeding, grooming, and hygiene tasks.
- Eye-hand coordination, such as throwing and catching a ball and drawing shapes.
- Visual perceptual skills.
- Graphomotor skills, from the basics of letter formation to taking notes in class.
- Social skills and play skills.

• Assistive technology needs like molded pencil grips and slant boards, access methods for computers and communication devices, use of wheelchairs, and adaptive equipment like reachers and dressing aids for clients with physical disabilities.

With such a broad range of practice areas, it's no wonder every OT does not have in-depth knowledge and expertise in the area of sensory processing. Some focus on orthopedic rehabilitation, fine motor and graphomotor skills, and so on. When helping kids and teens with sensory problems, be sure to collaborate with an OT who incorporates a sensory integrative frame of reference (OT-SI) and has training and experience in pediatric sensory processing assessment and intervention.

EVALUATION AND TREATMENT

The starting point is an initial assessment in the form of functional tests, clinical observations, and caregiver interviews. Caregiver or self questionnaires such as those discussed in Chapter 4 may be used. In addition to evaluating responses within each sensory system plus multisensory integration abilities, the OT will assess factors such as range of motion, muscle tone and strength, postural control and movement patterns, eye-hand coordination, and motor planning skills. A comprehensive OT evaluation will also assess fine motor, handwriting, visual perceptual, and self-care skills, and more. Ideally, the OT will also observe the child outside of the evaluation arena to see how he functions at home, at school, and out and about in the community.

While occupational therapy is individualized to each client's needs, the underlying premise is always that the nervous system can be rewired to work more efficiently thanks to neural plasticity. The basic tenet of neuroscience applies equally to occupational, physical, and even psychotherapy: Nerves that fire together wire together—and the more often they fire together, the more quickly and effectively they'll wire together. Therefore, sensory integrative treatment provides thoughtfully designed, repeated stimulation of multisensory systems graded relative to the child's tolerance and skill level. In other words, OT-SI treatment is a blast.

OT-SI therapy is typically provided in a specially designed setting sometimes called a sensory gym that has equipment such as swings, ladders, tunnels, scooters, trampolines, and ball pits. In a sensory gym, the child works one on one with an OT who purposefully engineers the environment in a way that promotes exploration and challenge and minimizes obstacles to success. The child and OT collaborate on ideas and activity choices, and the child actively engages in activities that are set up to provide the just-right challenge.

Occupational therapist Markus Jarrow, clinical director of the SMILE Center in New York City, writes:

> In treatment, you may see your child flying and spinning through space on swings hanging from the ceiling. You may see her climbing over or under enormous padded obstacles, up rope ladders or through suspended tunnels. She may zip by you on a scooter board, holding tight to a bungee cord, or jump from a platform into a crash mat or ball pit.
>
> Treatment with another child may appear completely different . . . at least initially. You may see him sitting with the clinician in a dimly lit room, wearing a pressure garment, covered in heavy blankets attending to an activity. You may see him gently rocking on a swing with the clinician cradling him from behind, or slowly rolling over a soft surface to the rhythmical hum of the therapist. He may be sitting quietly in a dark corner, blowing bubbles through a hose with headphones on. SI treatment can appear very different from one child to the next as it is individualized to each child's unique sensory needs. While an experienced clinician can make treatment simply look fun and playful, rest assured careful clinical reasoning is behind every move. (Jarrow, 2010, pp. 269–270)

Not all OT treatment occurs in a sensory gym. Home-based OT promotes sensory exploration, learning, and integration in the child's familiar space using the child's own toys, seating, stairs, and any equipment needed to help the child. At home, a parent may see the child sitting on a bolster batting at a balloon suspended from the ceiling, jumping on a mini trampoline while identifying foam letters as they zoom by, listening to special music over headphones while standing on a balance board, or playing barefoot in a bin full of dry rice and beans. You may see a child writing with her finger on a table-top covered with chocolate pudding while bouncing gently on a large therapy ball.

Parents and other caregivers can be shown firsthand how to help the child overcome sensory obstacles that cause friction, such as how to provide tactile desensitization prior to and deep pressure while washing a young child's hair, how to arrange a school-age child's room with sensory-friendly seating and lighting for homework, and how to provide a teenager with vestibular input that satisfies his need to move prior to sitting down at the dinner table.

The OT can train and closely monitor parents, babysitters, teachers, and other clinicians and caregivers as they implement sensory interventions such as the deep pressure proprioceptive touch protocol (more commonly known as brushing), astronaut training (a vestibular-visual-auditory protocol), sound-based therapy programs, and other recommended therapeutic exercises and activities.

At home, in a residential care facility, school, or other setting, the OT should assess the environment and help the family and other caregivers to modify it as necessary. For example, a child who has sleep difficulties may benefit from adding room-darkening, sound-dampening curtains, a white noise machine, and a soft, body-conforming pillow-top mattress cover on top of a hard mattress. The OT may help caregivers to recognize that the client is visually sensitive and may be struggling with grooming and hygiene tasks because she is avoiding the fluorescent lighting in the bathroom—and may give advice on changing the light fixture, adding a different source of illumination, or having the child engage in these tasks in a different room altogether.

The OT should help the family integrate sensory strategies into daily life, such as having an older child push the baby's stroller for proprioceptive input, or having him sit on a T-stool or low bench rather than melting into the couch while watching TV, jump on his mini-trampoline for 5 minutes prior to tabletop work, or use an inflated "wiggle cushion" to move while seated, as discussed in Chapter 6.

The OT who treats a child in the home will likely incorporate developmental and rehabilitative approaches as well, helping clients with tasks such as hair and body care, tying shoelaces, doing puzzles and mazes, handwriting and keyboarding, and simple meal preparation for older kids.

Some children receive school-based occupational therapy services through the school district (see Chapter 7). In school settings, OT services must enable the student to access the educational curriculum rather than addressing sensory issues only. Sensory smart school-based OTs recognize that kids experiencing problems at school frequently have underlying sensory processing challenges. A student may not be able to sit still in class for reasons such as low muscle tone and limited core strength, impaired body awareness, poor vestibular processing, or learning disabilities and anxiety. The child who dawdles on the stairs and in hallways and is therefore constantly late to class and in trouble may have trouble with depth perception, postural insecurity, and poor spatial orientation. Some schools—especially those with a significant number of students on the autism spectrum—do have facilities and equipment for providing sensory-based interventions but others do not and will refer out. Finally, keep in mind that some school-based therapists and school staff—especially in schools that do not have special education students—are not well versed in sensory processing issues and focus entirely on end results such as academics and behavior.

SENSORY PROGRAMS

Whether the child receives therapy at a sensory gym, at home, or at school, and no matter how marvelous the OT is or how frequent treatment sessions are, therapy is not real life, which occurs 24 hours a day, 7 days a week. This is why family members, caregivers, and school staff need to get involved with what OTs have historically called a sensory diet, a term coined by OT Patricia Wilbarger (Wilbarger, 1984). Since most people think of food when they hear the term "diet," the term "sensory program" may help to avoid such confusion.

Just as parents wouldn't consider waiting until dinnertime to meet a child's daily nutritional needs, they shouldn't wait until the child's therapy appointment to meet sensory needs. A sensory program is a personalized schedule of activities that help the child feel satisfied all day long, so she's not seeking sensation because she's starved for input or withdrawn and stimming because she's in sensory overload. The goal is to give the child the right type of sensory input in regular, controlled doses so there's no need to resort to unwanted behaviors. Instead of bulldozing into siblings to get deep pressure input, the child can crash into a safely arranged "crash pad." Instead of chewing on a pencil, chair leg, or hand, the student can chomp on a safe, age-appropriate oral chewy. Engaging in well-planned, sensory-rich input throughout the day helps balance arousal levels, reinforces new neural pathways in the brain and body, and helps the child be increasingly comfortable and functional in everyday life.

In addition to therapeutically beneficial exercises and activities, a sensory program should include environmental and task modifications that enable the child or teen to better participate in his life daily life occupations. These may include many of the strategies discussed in Chapters 6 and 7 such as changing lighting, seating, clothing, body care products, and more.

A sensory program must be tailored for each client. Personalized recommendations may include activities and modifications such as these:

- Wake-up time: Hugs, massage, deep-pressure brushing, playing activating music, taking a shower with a pleasant-smelling body wash and scrubby, eating protein for breakfast rather than pure carbohydrates.
- Before school: Dance, jump, take stairs instead of elevator, ride bicycle or scooter to school.
- Arrival at school: Arrive early to avoid the overcrowded school lobby, take quiet time with a book, or run around the gym or yard to burn off steam.
- Frequent breaks: Sensory "snacks" such as jumping jacks, wall push-ups, a quick run, or a break from high stimulation by going into a dimly lit, quiet area.
- Lunchtime: Engage in movement activities before sitting down to eat; suck on a mint or sour ball to "wake up" the mouth prior to eating.

- Special classes such as art, music, and gym: Wear noise-reducing earphones, inhale favored essential oils to mask unpleasant odors, massage hands to desensitize prior to handling messy materials.

- After school: Assess and select activities that satisfy the child's need for quiet down time or to burn off suppressed energy.

- Homework time: Sit on a ball chair or inflatable seat cushion, use a hand fidget, chew gum, clear desk surface of all extraneous objects, use nonglare tabletop lighting.

- Dinner time: Engage in intense vestibular activities prior to sitting down, help carry plates and platters to table, use utensils with built-up handles for easy grip, place small portions on plate to avoid visual overload.

- Bedtime: Begin bedtime routine one hour prior; begin with rough-housing play, warm bath, back and foot massage, reading.

- Sleep time: Use a heavy blanket, soft pajamas and bed linens, white noise machine, night light or darkness as preferred.

Again, these are just generic examples of a sensory diet. What will work best varies from person to person. And while routines and consistency are helpful, remember that as the child's needs change, sensory diet strategies will need to change too.

PTS, SLPS, SEITS, AND MORE

Depending on the child's issues, she may receive "related services" such as physical therapy, speech-language therapy, or have a special education itinerant teacher (SEIT) or other specialized instruction through early intervention, the school system, or privately. While an increasing number of these professionals are becoming more familiar with the concept of sensory processing, the PT, speech-language pathologist (SLP), or SEIT treating the child may not be at all knowledgeable about how to deal with sensory issues. All of them will need to learn about the particular child's sensory challenges and how that impacts their area of expertise. Collaboration between all of these professionals along with OTs and mental health clinicians can make a big difference.

For example, kids with low muscle tone and poor body awareness typically have poor postural control and a weak diaphragm and
accessory respiratory muscles. This results in shallow breathing and
poor oxygenation. A common technique is to instruct a child who
is becoming upset or panicked to stop and breathe before reacting.
As a result, the child may breathe quickly and superficially, causing
counterproductive hyperventilation. Working collaboratively, the OT
can provide supportive seating and, along with the PT, strengthen
core musculature including the muscles needed for erect posture
and respiration, facilitating the respiratory control needed to speak
articulately in speech therapy and to use calming deep breathing to
regulate emotions and behavior in counseling.

All team members need to learn the importance of movement and
that the best results never come from having a child sit in a chair
and work at a table for hours. The OT can teach team members how
to use vestibular stimulation to increase speech production, explaining that the vestibular system and the cochlea (the adjacent hearing portion of the inner ear) are anatomically and physiologically
connected, sharing fluids and even some of the same nerve fibers.
Research shows that vestibular stimulation can increase sponta-
neous vocalization (Ray, King, & Grandin, 1988; Schueli, Henn, &
Brugger, 1999). Thus the OT may suggest that the child engage
in movement activities prior to or during therapy such as jumping
on a trampoline, using a swing or jump rope, stretching muscles,
changing her head position by log rolling or touching her toes, or at
the very least sitting on a ball chair and gently bouncing if tabletop
tasks are required.

Physical Therapists

PTs address neuromuscular and orthopedic conditions including
limited mobility and range of motion, gait deviations, poor muscle
tone, strength, endurance, motor coordination and planning, musculoskeletal pain, and more. PTs who work with children should understand how deficits in sensory processing result in difficulty using
sensory feedback loops needed to guide movements.

Consider descending stairs. You can probably do so without even thinking since you rely on ingrained motor plans based on sensory feedback from your visual, vestibular, and proprioceptive systems. To help a child learn to descend stairs safely and efficiently, the PT will work on strengthening muscles and repeating the movement pattern until it becomes a permanent motor plan. The PT needs to recognize that underlying sensory issues may interfere with the development of this motor plan and may prevent the child from descending stairs at a reasonable, safe pace. The child with impaired depth perception, for example, is unable to use visual feedback to guide his neuromuscular efforts, for example, looking at the next step, gauging how far he needs to step, and appropriately activating the right muscles. Instead he relies on tactile input, feeling around in space with his foot to locate the next step. Hopefully he is not distracted by the sensation of his shoes and socks or the feeling of the bannister. Poor vestibular processing may impact his ability to maintain his balance while impaired proprioception may interfere with sensing when his entire foot is planted firmly on the step surface, making him unstable, unsafe, and often unwilling to persist with such a task.

Speech-Language Pathologists

SLPs address receptive and expressive language, articulation, pragmatic (social) language, auditory processing difficulties, and oral-motor problems such as weakness of the tongue, lips, and jaw that may interfere with speech production, eating, and swallowing. Some SLPs specialize in feeding therapy, as do some OTs (see Chapter 6 for information on when to refer to a feeding specialist).

It is important that SLPs understand how sensory issues affect their clients. A child who has oral tactile hypersensitivity may need oral tactile desensitization using tools such as Den-Tips and oral vibrators in and around the mouth. If she has low oral muscle tone and does not process oral sensations well, she may benefit from alerting tools such as ice pops and sour or spicy treats. Increasing oral sensory awareness will help the child to coordinate the many muscles of the mouth and process when she is drooling, pocketing food in her cheeks, and so on.

Of course, the SLP needs to know if the child has auditory sensory issues, as this will directly impact how speech-language therapy services are delivered. The SLP may need to use a perky, high-pitched tone of voice with a hyposensitive, low-arousal client and a lower, deeper voice for a child who is sensitive to high-pitched voices. For a child with SPD, working in a group on speech and language issues—as often occurs in schools—may be contraindicated.

SEITs, Behavior Analysts, and Others

Children who are struggling in general education classrooms may be eligible for SEIT services in the home, daycare, or school to address cognitive development and learning issues. Paraprofessionals and "shadows" may also be brought in to help the student get engaged, stay on task, and remain safe in school.

When behavior is a major problem, a behaviorist may be engaged, typically for intensive treatment over many hours per session. Behavioral analysis is confined to modifying observable behaviors that interfere with learning and excludes subjective experiences such as emotions or motivation. Traditionally, board-certified behavior analysts and board-certified assistant behavior analysts have been taught that sensory processing issues are not real and that sensory treatments are unproven, and were specifically instructed not to endorse or address sensory processing difficulties (Behavior Analyst Certification Board, 2011). Fortunately, many behavior analysts are recognizing how very real and oftentimes disabling sensory issues are and have learned to collaborate with OTs and others to ensure that their clients' sensory challenges are minimized in order to maximize their behavioral interventions.

Sensory issues should never, ever be ignored, regardless of the kind of educational or behavioral program the child attends. After all, if the child is uncomfortable or in pain, not getting the sensory input he needs or overwhelmed by demands to process sensory input simultaneously, he will be unable to fully benefit from everyone's best-intentioned efforts.

Developmental Optometrists and Other Vision Specialists

Remember that a child with vision deficits sees the world in his own way and doesn't realize others see things any differently. Many children with visual processing difficulties have undiagnosed vision problems. While a quick vision screening at a pediatrician's office or at school can be helpful, it is by no means a vision evaluation. An eye exam in the pediatrician's office is a simple screening that tests whether a child can see in both eyes at one distance. It does not test for farsightedness, eye disease, or visual skills such as eye teaming, tracking, or near-to-far refocusing.

The American Optometric Association recommends vision exams by qualified vision care professionals. The first eye exam should be between the age of 6 months and one year, the second exam before entering kindergarten, and then annually. Children at high risk for the development of eye and vision problems due to developmental delays, high refractive error, prematurity or low birth weight, seizures, or other central nervous system dysfunction should have their eyes evaluated more often.

A pediatric ophthalmologist is a medical doctor who specializes in the diagnosis and treatment of eye disease using surgical and medical methods. For example, the ophthalmologist will thoroughly assess eye health and visual acuity, prescribe eyeglasses if needed, perform surgeries such as removing cataracts and correcting ocular misalignment such as strabismus, and medically manage eye diseases such as glaucoma, macular degeneration, and diabetic retinopathy.

A doctor of optometry also examines, diagnoses, treats, and manages diseases, injuries, and disorders of the eye and the visual system but does not perform eye surgery. A developmental optometrist, also called a behavioral optometrist, has obtained additional training in the development and use of functional vision including binocular vision, depth perception, eye movements, and visual deficits. The developmental optometrist may prescribe eyeglasses or may use special lenses such as yoked prism lenses and optometric vision therapy to nonsurgically alter the way a person's visual system works. Developmental optometrists can work closely with the treatment team for the child or teen with visual sensory issues, recommending strategies such as sitting close to the front of the room, using enlarged typefaces on worksheets and other printed matter, and prescribing eye strengthening exercises to be done in their office, at home, or in OT sessions. A good place to find a qualified developmental optometrist is through the College of Optometrists in Vision Development (covd.org).

Audiologists

An audiologist who is knowledgeable about sensory issues knows that a child may pass a standard hearing test with flying colors but can still have auditory deficits. Difficulties with hypersensitivity or hyperacusis, over- or undersensitivity to particular sound frequencies, discriminating between relevant voices and superfluous background noises, and other auditory issues may make listening difficult in many environments. The audiologist may then recommend auditory strategies and interventions such as having the student sit near the teacher, providing written directions to supplement auditory instructions, and using an FM Unit at school or work. This device consists of a transmitter placed near or worn by the speaker (usually a teacher) and a receiver placed near or worn by the listener that raises the speaker's voice above background noise (technically, it enhances the signal-to-noise ratio).

The audiology exam should include the following:

- Testing for sensitivity to a wide spectrum of frequency ranges.
- The lowest decibel level heard, ideally beginning with a level of volume not typically detected by the human ear, such as negative 15 decibels.
- Tympanogram to check for fluid in the ears.
- Speech discrimination skills.

Ear, Nose, and Throat Doctors, Allergists, and Nutritionists

A common cause of auditory problems due to ear structure difficulties is middle ear infections that result in collection of fluid behind
the eardrums, also known as effusions. Nearly one in six school-age
children has an auditory problem severe enough to cause learning
challenges, with effusions being the most common cause of hearing
impairment, according to Drs. Fernette and Brock Eide (Eide & Eide,
2006, pp. 115–117). The Eides explain that effusions dampen sound
transmission in the middle ear, causing an average hearing loss of 25
decibels. At this level of hearing loss, a student may miss 30–50 percent of what the teacher says. Most effusions take about 40 days to
drain. A student who gets frequent ear infections and resulting effusions will experience hearing loss and resulting auditory processing
and learning challenges during much of the school year.

Middle ear effusions are generally caused by eustachian tube dysfunction due to enlarged tonsils or adenoids or allergies. The student
who suffers from frequent ear infections should be seen by an ear,
nose, and throat doctor. The child should also be seen by an allergist,
who can test for food and environmental allergies that may be contributing to the ear infections, chronic sinus infections, gastric disturbances, and more.

Allergies don't just impact the ears, sinuses, and belly. The body's
immune system responds to foreign pathogens (allergens) by producing histamines that trigger an inflammatory response by dilating blood
vessels, which of course are virtually all over the body. Symptoms of
histamine reaction include swelling, redness, skin rash, hives, itching,
headaches, and respiratory distress. A child with extremely sensitive
skin may be profoundly relieved when an unknown allergen is identified and removed from the environment and a chronic histamine
reaction is alleviated. The most common environmental allergens are
dust, pollen, animal dander, mold, mites, and insect bites. The most
common food allergens are peanuts, tree nuts, dairy products, wheat,
shellfish, eggs, and soy.

A person may undergo the standard battery of allergy tests and be told there's nothing wrong. Yet sensory issues may get worse at a certain time of year (such as springtime hay fever season or autumn when damp leaves get moldy) or when the child eats certain foods. This is because the child is experiencing an environmental or food intolerance rather than a full-fledged allergic reaction.

Additional food response tests can identify offending foods. A parent or caregiver can also try food elimination, removing a suspected food for two weeks, assessing changes at home and at school, and then slowly reintroducing the food, again looking for any changes. It will be very important to communicate about this with all caregivers and therapists so that everyone can avoid giving the child the questionable food and monitor the child's response.

Nutritionists can play a key role in identifying foods that are not well tolerated as well as adding foods that will bolster the child's immune system and build the child's brain and body from the inside out. After all, what we ingest creates the biochemical substrates for every cell in the body and sets up the ability to respond—or not—to therapy.

A child who eats well feels well and functions better. This is easier said than done for kids who are picky eaters and problem feeders. A nutritionist can work hand in hand with parents, feeding therapists, OTs, and others to come up with a workable nutritional program that includes supplements such as multivitamins and essential fatty acids that can help correct imbalances, boost cellular growth, and normalize transmission between nerve cell fibers to facilitate cognitive, motor, and sensory function.

Nutritionist Kelly Dorfman, author of *Cure Your Child With Food*, is a nutrition detective who helps people with complex ailments and symptoms ranging from chronic bad moods to gastric disturbances to sleep problems. Dorfman described a 4-year-old referred to her by an OT:

> This child could not be touched by anyone and screamed a lot. His tactile sensitivity was so bad that the OT could not get near enough to do therapy. He was very thin because his tactile defensiveness limited him to eating just a few foods—mainly dry cereal, bread,

and waffles. He had no fruit, vegetables or protein sources. He was literally so nutritionally deficient that he could not be worked with in therapy. The family and I decided to close the gap between what he was willing to eat and what he needed to eat for his neurological development using a potent, custom-made vitamin and mineral supplement which we were able to flavor like medicine he'd accepted in the past. We also compounded it into an unflavored oil that could be drizzled lightly on his waffles. Within a few weeks of taking the supplements, the OT was able to approach him and he quickly began to improve. (Dorfman, personal communication, October 14, 2012)

Developmental Pediatricians

A developmental pediatrician, sometimes called a developmental-behavioral pediatrician, is a medical doctor who is board certified in pediatrics and has additional subspecialty training. These specially trained pediatricians work with children and adolescents with a wide range of developmental and behavioral difficulties in settings such as hospitals, rehabilitation centers, and private practice.

Some developmental pediatricians are happy to collaborate as part of the treatment team. At the very least, the family should be encouraged to share evaluations and recommendations from the developmental pediatrician with all team members.

Other Complementary Therapies

Children with sensory processing issues may find some help from complementary therapies such as craniosacral therapy, massage therapy, chiropractic, homeopathy, and other approaches. Encourage families and clients to share when they are using such services so that you can monitor their impact on how your client seems to feel and function. For example, you may find that your client is significantly more relaxed for several days following a deep tissue massage from a licensed professional. If so, you may want to encourage massage on a regular basis.

The child, teen, or young adult you are treating as a clinician may well also be working with another professional discussed in this chapter. Parents may not be forthcoming about this simply because they may not realize how important the big picture is or how some approaches can be contraindicated. For example, if the child reacts badly to sweets, candy shouldn't be used as a reward in therapy sessions. If a child is able to focus and attend if he moves, he should not be forced to sit motionless for an hour.

Whenever possible, attend at least one treatment session with the child's other clinicians. This will help you to have a better sense of the people influencing the child's world and give you a chance to learn more about his strengths and weaknesses. It will also give you an opportunity to communicate strategies you know are helpful. You may request to be alerted by phone, e-mail, or letter of any changes in intervention that may impact your treatments. In all, the more fully rounded your understanding of the child's world, the better you will be able to help.

CHAPTER 6

Empowering Strategies
for Parents

Sensory processing challenges can bewilder even the most confident, competent parent. The mother of three may not understand why her infant arches his back and wails whenever she attempts to hold him. A father may not understand why it takes his darling daughter 2 hours of tears, begging, and screaming to get ready for school. A child who is on the move from the moment he wakes up until he goes to bed, jumping from toy to toy, climbing like an incautious little monkey on furniture, banging into other children on the playground, can be simply exhausting.

Many parents first learn about SPD when they seek help because their child is not meeting developmental milestones like crawling or speaking on schedule. For others, sensory problems may not be apparent until the child starts school; the placid toddler who is comfortable and happy at home may become overwhelmed by the sights, sounds, and activity of the classroom coupled with increased behavioral and academic expectations.

Parents may walk away from a developmental evaluation with the dreaded but perhaps anticipated diagnosis of a fine motor, gross motor, or speech delay or something even more serious such as autism or attention disorder, plus the mystifying diagnosis of SPD.

When parents first learn that their child is not developing typically, it is terribly distressing, to say the least. Even if there is only a sensory processing problem with no additional diagnosis, parents may be anxious and confused. What does this mean for the child's future? Will she fail miserably in school? Will he eventually make friends? Will daily life always be a struggle? Did they do something to cause this condition? Can they fix their child?

Sometimes the very symptoms pinpointed as problematic—such as oversensitivity to certain sounds and textures—may be something the parents also experience, so it seems perfectly normal. The apple often doesn't fall far from the tree. The world that we perceive is, simply, our world.

All parents benefit from compassionate reassurance. Fortunately, today there are effective interventions and plenty of practical strategies and tools that will empower them to understand and help their children overcome their challenges.

SET THE CHILD UP FOR SUCCESS

Parenting a child with sensory issues means scheduling in extra time, cultivating some extra patience, and being both flexible and creative. While every child is different, the following strategies will help most kids with sensory problems.

Increase Predictability and Control

Children who struggle with sensory issues don't always receive accurate, reliable information about their bodies and their place in the world and thrive on predictability and having a sense of control over their lives. While most children love familiarity such as having the same favorite bedtime book read to them night after night, most SPD children absolutely require predictability to avoid becoming overaroused or anxious.

It may help to provide verbal or a visual schedule so the child knows what to expect and can better tolerate transitions between activities. A child may have difficulty getting everything done before school. A morning schedule could look like this, with items checked off as they are completed:

- 7:00 a.m. Wake up.
  - Engage in morning sensory diet activities (list these).
  - Brush teeth, wash face, comb hair.
  - Get dressed.
  - Put backpack by front door.
  - Eat breakfast.
  - Put dishes in the dishwasher.
- 8:15 a.m. Get on bus.

If a parent has a lot of errands to run after she picks up the child from school, she and the child can review a written schedule. The parent can draw pictures or attach photos if the child does not yet read. These should then be reviewed together, emphasizing sequence, before the child goes to school. "After school, we will go to the dry cleaner, then the supermarket, then the post office, and then we'll go to the playground for one hour."

A child may benefit from a written or visual after-school checklist:

- 3:00 p.m. Pick up from school.
  - Snack
  - Dry cleaner
  - Supermarket
  - Post office
  - Playground
- 5:30 p.m. Written homework
- 6:30 p.m. Dinner
- 7:30 p.m. Reading homework
- 8:30 p.m. Shower
- 9:00 p.m. Bedtime

Avoid Overscheduling

If a child is overwhelmed by too many transitions from one activity to another, parents should avoid planning too many errands, and consider whether going to the playground first would actually enable the child to better tolerate the agenda, ultimately saving time, trouble, and headache in terms of managing unwanted behavioral reactions.

Give Fair Warning

Kids with sensory issues often have difficulty shifting from one activity to another. Because they are so distracted by sensations, it may take them a while to settle into a task and then, just when they are close to finished building a block tower or coloring a picture of My Little Pony, it's time to stop.

Teach parents, teachers, and others to let kids know they have 30 minutes to play or work on a project, then give them 15-minute, 10-minute, and 5-minute warnings. Because children have a notoriously poor sense of time, a timer may help. Beware of timers with sounds that are too jarring, or the child may wind up losing time because he is anxious about the impending noise. A visual timer such as the Time Timer works best for many kids (see page 209). This timer, which can be set for up to 1 hour, has a red, round disk that slowly shrinks as time elapses.

Provide Acceptable Choices

Parents can give children a needed sense of control by providing some options. At dinner, rather than telling the child she must eat some vegetables, the parent can offer a choice of broccoli or sugar snap peas. Brushing teeth is not a choice, but a parent can provide two flavors of toothpaste.

Break Up Large Tasks

Long or complicated processes should be broken into manageable units. Doing homework is mandatory, but a parent can help a child manage multiple, lengthy assignments by breaking them up into reasonable chunks such as doing the math work, having a snack, then science, then dinner, and then reading after dessert. A child may be much more compliant about cleaning her room if a parent prompts her to put all of her clothes in the hamper and all of the books on the shelf instead of insisting that she "clean up this mess *right now!*"

Provide Needed Sensory Input

For a child with sensory problems, being hungry for sensory input can spell disaster. Sensory activities that help the child feel good and function well are essential. Kids who are overaroused will benefit from calming, soothing activities such as getting a quick massage or back rub, playing with some Silly Putty, wearing a weighted vest, or sitting quietly in a softly lit room. Kids who are underaroused may benefit from activating tasks such as jumping on a mini trampoline, dancing to peppy music, and so on. For more on sensory diet activities please see Chapter 5.

Take a Break

As a culture, we stress productivity above all. There is a tendency to think we should be doing something at all times. We should work hard and play hard. Sometimes, we just need to *be*. We need to not be engaged in doing work, reading a book, surfing the Internet, checking e-mail, using the cell phone, cleaning up, doing laundry, or whatever. It's often in those quiet, meditative times that we find inner peace. Whether it's petting a cat or just watching the clouds go by, taking breaks often enables kids and adults to compose themselves and be at their best.

SENSORY PROBLEM OR BEHAVIOR PROBLEM?

Many parents, teachers, and even therapists struggle with telling the difference between what is caused by sensory issues and what is purely behavioral. The answer is seldom simple and almost always requires rethinking your ideas about behavior as well as some detective work.

It may help to think of behaviors simply as observable symptoms of something else. If you know the child has sensory issues, the best bet is to assume that the child's reactions are due to inability to cope with sensory processing demands rather than avoidant, manipulative, or attention-seeking behavior unless there is a compelling reason to think otherwise. Then you need to identify the sensory triggers and situations that result in negative behavioral reactions. So yes, the end result is behavioral, but it's behavior driven by underlying sensory problems.

Four Key Questions to Ask

The Sensory Screening Tool in Chapter 2 is designed to help parents and others to consider which experiences, situations, and tasks are especially difficult for the child. The following questions will help them to clarify their observations:

1. When did the reaction start? Is the behavior something the child has been doing for a long time, such as banging his head every time you go into a store? Or is it something new, such as suddenly swiping at his ears when there is a lot of noise around (which may indicate an ear infection)?

2. How predictable is the reaction? Are there certain situations that are consistently difficult? When was the last time it happened? Does the child always have a tantrum in all kinds of stores or just the toy store and just when she doesn't get something she wants? Does the child show up late for every class? Does he always avoid something he can't handle?

3. What and who are the triggers? Does the problem always occur around certain people? Does the child always misbehave around a certain teacher or therapist? Does one particular in-law seem to agitate the child? Is there one classroom subject that is always hard for the child, such as art or music?

4. What are the underlying hidden sensory demands? Consider what the challenges are for each sensory system. For example, taking a bath gives a lot of tactile input in terms of water pressure and temperature on the skin, room temperature, towel texture, shampoo and soap texture; smell of bathing products; sounds of water on porcelain tub in a room that echoes due to minimal sound-absorbing fabrics; typically bright fluorescent lighting and the need to close eyes during shampooing; balance issues while standing for a shower or sitting in the tub, especially with eyes closed, and so on. Any discomfort with one of these sensory experiences could make the entire bathing experience very difficult.

Keep a Behavior Journal

To help parents gain further insight into difficult situations and unwanted behaviors, it will help to have parents, teachers, and other caregivers keep a journal in order to clarify what is going on. It may well be that some of the peculiar or baffling behaviors actually occur in fairly predictable patterns.

Keeping a journal may help the parent of an older child recognize a correlation between increased sensory reactions when there is too much stimulation (or too little stimulation) in the form of overscheduling (or too much free time), or issues such as being tired, hungry, sick, or social or emotional factors. Some children's sensory issues worsen each spring and fall due to seasonal allergies. Some seem to cycle monthly, corresponding to menstrual cycles. Others are set off by school exams. Others are worse when the child eats fruit sprayed with pesticides or when the house has just been cleaned with harsh chemicals.

In a journal, have involved adults or capable teens note:

- Date, day of the week, and time of problematic behavior.
- Observed behavior, describing exactly what happened.
- Context of behavior: where it occurred and with whom as well as what was happening leading up to the event.
- All food and beverages—everything that goes into the mouth (note artificial sweeteners and food dyes and whether they are organic to rule out possible pesticides).
- Nutritional supplements.
- Medications and vaccinations.
- Health status, including allergy flare-ups, fevers, sinus problems, headaches.
- Weather, including barometric pressure, precipitation, and temperature.
- Social engagements (parties, holidays, dates).
- School and after-school activities: assemblies, special events, sports.
- Tests and other academic demands.

- Household cleaning products used.
- Menstrual periods, including cramps and bloating.
- Sleep habits—bedtime and wake-up time, quality of sleep, number of awakenings, naps.
- Bowel and bladder habits if known.

Ideally, the journal should be kept for at least one month or two to four weeks per season for a year to capture as much data as possible. While it is indeed a lot of work, keeping a journal, even if just for one week, can reveal invaluable insights and result in some wonderfully effective strategies.

Kevin, a 14-year-old with mild sensory issues and learning challenges, was generally a well-behaved, even-tempered child, but every week or two he would lose all ability to tolerate frustration and become completely irritable and impatient with his classmates, his little sister, and even the dog that he adored. While he had always been hypersensitive to sound and touch, this was not like him. The family, school psychologist, and OT were worried that he might be showing signs of bipolar disorder.

They were told to record everything. The team soon noticed that every time a low-pressure weather front came through, Kevin's over-the-top behavior started up as well. The nastiness would subside once the front passed. It also seemed that foods with refined sugars like doughnuts, cookies, cake, and candy, never great for him, were especially problematic during these times. While they obviously couldn't control the weather, they learned to reduce avoidable sensory demands and helped him gain insight into what was driving his behavior, which he felt terrible about.

Now Kevin has a barometer in his own room and a weather app showing barometric pressure on his computer at school so he can tell the team what's happening with the weather and take proactive steps at school and at home to keep himself from blowing up. He gets extra down time, doubles up on sensory activities that help him stay organized, and is careful to avoid sugary snacks during these periods. He is much more in control of himself now.

Temper Tantrums Versus Sensory Meltdowns

Let's consider so-called temper tantrums, all too common when young children are learning to manage their emotions and frustrations. Researchers have found that over 80 percent of preschoolers ages 3–5 have one or more tantrums in a month, but that fewer than 10 percent of young children have a daily temper tantrum (Wakschlag et al., 2012). Using a parent questionnaire called the Multidimensional Assessment of Preschool Disruptive Behavior (MAP-BP) to help quantify the frequency, quality, and severity of many temper tantrum behaviors as well as anger management abilities, the study found that:

- 61 percent of preschoolers threw tantrums when frustrated, angry, or upset.
- 58 percent threw tantrums during daily routines such as bedtime, mealtime, or getting dressed.
- While 56 percent threw tantrums with their parents, only 36 percent had tantrums with an adult such as a teacher or babysitter.
- 28 percent broke or destroyed objects and 24 percent hit, bit, or kicked somebody.
- Parents could not discern a reason for 26 percent of tantrums.

We know that the longer and more frequent tantrums are, the greater the likelihood that they are not developmentally typical and that something more serious is going on, especially in older children.

It is essential to differentiate between a temper tantrum due to emotional factors such as the child not getting what he desires and a sensory meltdown due to overstimulation in which neurobiological needs are not being met. The observable actions may be identical, but the root causes may be entirely different.

Sensory Meltdowns

- Mismatch between situation and sensory processing capability.
- Sensory needs are not being met.
- Sensory stimulation is uncomfortable or painful.

- Demands to manage responses to sensory input are overwhelming.
- May injure self or others as a result of fight-or-flight stress response.

Behavior Tantrums

- Mismatch between situation and emotional factors including cognition and coping skills.
- Emotional needs and desires are not being met.
- Need for attention is not being met.
- Generally will not injure self intentionally.

Child Acts Out in the Toy Store

Behavioral: Isabelle wants a new doll and Mom says no. She starts whining and if Mom does not relent she throws herself on the floor and starts to cry and yell. The last time this happened, Mom relented and bought the toy Isabelle wanted. It may well work again this time.

Sensory: Sofia has both auditory and visual sensitivities, so going into a toy store with noisy electronics, lots of people talking, plus aisles of colorful toys, is making her head buzz and she starts to feel shaky and spooked. She sees a doll she likes and asks Mommy to buy it. When Mom says no, it's too much for her to deal with. She throws herself on the floor and starts to cry and yell. She just can't help herself.

Child Acts Out at the Dinner Table

Behavioral: Justin is building with his Legos. He is not especially hungry and he doesn't like what's for dinner either. He takes a few bites because his parents make him and then gets up to go play. He can always snack on something later. When his father insists that he remain at the table even if he is done eating, he picks up his plate and throws it on the floor. His father sends him to his room for a time-out.

Sensory: Jake has low muscle tone and poor proprioceptive processing skills. He hates sitting at the dinner table because he isn't comfortable in his chair and sometimes falls out of it, which makes his sister laugh at him. It's better for him to stand up while he is eating, and even better if he runs around the couch between bites. When his fed-up parents demand that he sit down and stay down, he picks up his plate and throws it on the floor. He father sends him to his room.

Always Late to Class

Behavioral: Rodney is a good student, but consistently shows up for class at least 10 minutes late. He walks friends to their classes and then realizes he forgot his textbook in his locker, so he needs to go there too. Math and science are boring and he rarely does his homework. If he goes late, they'll send him to the principal's office, which is fine with him. This way he won't get today's homework assignment and won't have to do it. He's been told that despite his good grades, he will not pass this semester if he continues with this bad attitude.

Sensory: David is a good student, but consistently shows up for class at least 10 minutes late. He just can't deal with the chaos between classes. He walks more slowly than his classmates and gets upset if he is jostled by others. He goes to a bathroom stall after each period and waits until the hall is clear before going to his next class. When told that he must be punctual getting to his classes, he says he just can't help it. He's been told that despite his good grades, he will not pass this semester if he continues with this bad attitude.

Having sensory problems does not give a child permission to misbehave. But it is essential to determine whether a parent, teacher or other person is punishing a child for a reaction that he cannot yet control. Parents, teachers, and others, including the child as he matures, need to become vigilant about predicting difficult situations, recognizing early warning signs of an impending meltdown, having a bag of tricks to circumvent the meltdown, and having a positive plan of action for when the child falls apart.

AN OUNCE OF PREVENTION

Most parents and clinicians frequently ask themselves: When should I push this child forward so that she gets used to daily life sensory experiences (taking her to the supermarket in the hope that repeated exposure will desensitize her)? When should I protect him entirely (such as never going to a supermarket)? To what degree should I accommodate his sensitivities (going to the supermarket during off hours for just a quick trip, letting him wear noise-canceling headphones)? This is not an easy dilemma to sort through, and it is one of the great challenges of raising a child with sensory processing issues, not to mention one who also happens to have several other developmental challenges.

When a child feels physically or emotionally distressed by sensory experiences, she cannot function at her best. If a child is truly uncomfortable or in pain, it's best to keep all three options in your mind. Yes, you do want her to be able to tolerate all kinds of experiences eventually; yes, you do want to avoid situations that she is simply unable to tolerate yet; and yes, it's a good idea to accommodate her sensitivities so that she can function at her best right now.

Recognize the Early Warning Signs

Once a child is pushed past the breaking point, it's virtually impossible to pull back. That's why it's so important to read the signs foreshadowing a problem that needs attention. Does the child start to get quiet? Speak more rapidly? Does the child start to physically withdraw? Become clingy? Does he start to engage in self-stimulatory behaviors? Does she become pale or flushed? Does he start to breathe rapidly or have an increased heart rate?

Always Have a Bag of Tricks

The sensory program strategies discussed in Chapter 5 are key ingredients in your plan to avert sensory meltdowns. By providing regulating sensory input at key points throughout the day—before school, before meals, standing in line, waiting in a doctor's office, while doing homework—you are enabling that child's nervous system to withstand the inevitable demands of daily life. Remember that old cliché: A stitch in time saves nine. Just taking a break can often save a situation. Taking several breaks during several hours' worth of homework, having a snack before after-school errands, doing some jumping jacks or running around the block before visiting Grandma, or chewing gum before sitting down for dinner can make a huge difference. If you know movement organizes your child, give him a choice of several movement activities you know he enjoys. If you know your child does well if she has something to do with her hands, make sure you bring along a busy bag with some squeeze balls and some crayons and a notepad.

> My 4½-year-old daughter has a lot of sensory problems. She's been completely potty trained for over a year now, but she began wetting herself at school because she refused to use the toilet. We thought it was because she might have separation anxiety and the school even talked about the possibility of oppositional defiant disorder. I finally got her to talk about it. The problem was she hated the way the paper towels feel and knew if she used the toilet she'd be forced to wash her hands and dry them with those paper towels. I sent in terrycloth towels from home and she started using the toilet at school. (Erin M., mother of a preschooler)

HANDLING AN ACTUAL MELTDOWN

Once a child is in sensory overload, the key is to save face and stay safe. It's usually counterproductive to try talking the child down intellectually when she is in the middle of a meltdown. Instead, the parent needs to defuse the situation.

Teach parents that if possible, they should remove the child to a location with a preferable level of sensory stimulation: a nice quiet spot with dim lighting and no foot traffic. The child can listen to soothing music over headphones, hold a comfort object, drink some water, or just breathe. Some firm pressure such as a back rub or cuddling may be in order, but only if the child welcomes it. Remember that taking a well-timed sensory retreat is quite different from a punishment or banishment. It's a chance to unload the bad feelings so the child can feel and function better.

Certainly a parent can and should talk about what happened afterward. Something as basic as, "I saw that you were having a really hard time. What do you think caused it? Do you think it was too crowded, noisy, smelly, or something there? Do you have some ideas about what we can do next time we're in a situation like that? I have some ideas you might like too." If the parent realizes she could have handled it differently herself, she can apologize. "I know going to the mall is hard for you. You did a great job until I made you go to too many stores. I'm sorry. I should have remembered that you need a break or that we should have returned another day. We'll do better to prevent what happened next time."

It can be very frustrating to be constantly dealing with a child's sensory issues when a parent is trying to get through a busy day, especially if other children are vying for attention. If the parent loses his temper and yells, he should wait until everyone has calmed down to talk about it. Spanking is never, ever an acceptable means of discipline. First, it teaches kids to communicate with their hands, which is not a good thing. Second, the sensation may be magnified; an oversensitive child may perceive a light swat as a frightening assault while an undersensitive child may think it's just super.

As with anything else, knowledge is power. As parents become more adept at predicting which situations will be difficult for the child, and everyone gets more accustomed to using sensory strategies that prevent problems in the first place, life with a sensory challenged child becomes less . . . challenging.

STRATEGIES FOR HANDLING DAILY LIFE TASKS

While some sensitive children become independent in tasks such as brushing their teeth and getting dressed early on, many others find such daily life tasks quite repellent. Scratchy hairbrush bristles, stinky shampoo, bubbling toothpaste, and more may result in early morning battles with parents trying to get the child clean, dressed, and out the door to school.

Parents may know that taking their child to a supermarket at 5 p.m. after a full day of school and after-school activities is a recipe for disaster and may gear their day to avoid doing this. Other trigger situations are harder to avoid. Holiday gatherings, getting ready for school, and going to the doctor are all events that can be extremely trying for parent and child alike.

Parenting children with sensory challenges usually requires a different set of rules than the ones the parents were raised with or what is recommended in parenting magazines. The parenting goals may still be the same, but the journey of raising happy, healthy, well-behaved children may take parents down roads they weren't aware even existed. Dealing with sensory issues takes extra compassion and lots of creative problem solving. In our book, *Raising a Sensory Smart Child*, Nancy Peske and I provided nearly 50 pages of practical solutions for everyday problems for parents and teachers that you may want to share. In the rest of this chapter you'll find strategies for the scenarios parents are most likely to need help with during your therapy sessions together.

As with everything sensory, the overarching principles are to assess the underlying issues, to determine what can and needs to be changed, and to increase the child's capacity to handle a wider variety of experiences. Let's consider a child who becomes very agitated when it comes to brushing his teeth. Ask:

1. What are the sensory demands that the child cannot tolerate? It is essential to do an activity analysis of problematic tasks or experiences, breaking them down into their sensory components. Is the toothbrush hurting the child's gums? Is it the taste or smell of the toothpaste? Does the toothpaste foam feel weird in the mouth? Is the child afraid of gagging on the foam? If you are able to determine what sensory aspect is problematic, is it something you can change or is it something the child must learn to deal with?

2. What about environmental context? Is the bathroom conducive to tooth brushing for this child? Is the fluorescent lighting too bright or flickering? Does the tiled bathroom echo too much? Would it help to add sound-absorbing materials such as a terrycloth shower curtain, fluffy towels, and a floor rug? Would the child do better in a different room? What can be changed in terms of environment, or is this a situation the child simply must learn to deal with?

3. Is the child feeling safe? Does standing on a step stool while brushing teeth at the sink make the child feel ungrounded and insecure?

Would the child do better sitting down? How can the child be helped to feel more physically and emotionally safe?

4. How can the child be better prepared for the activity? Is there a preparatory sensory activity that will help the child such as a quick, firm massage before brushing his teeth? Will it help the child to have the sequence of the steps spelled out verbally or in a written or picture list? Is he the kind of child who does better if he watches a video or reads a book about brushing teeth?

Problem-solving these situations becomes easier the more a parent tunes into the underlying issues and recognizes the strategies that will work best.

Face Washing

For children with tactile sensitivity, face washing can feel terrific or terrible. Here are some techniques to try:

• Experiment with different types of facial cleansers to find one with the right feel and scent. For example, a child may object to the feeling of soap bubbling up on the skin and prefer a nonlathering facial cleanser. Allow the child to smell different facial cleansers and select his favorite. Remember that bar soaps, foam pump soaps, liquid cleansers, and cleansing milks all present different tactile and smell experiences and it may take some trial and error to find a winner.

• Most sensitive people do better with firm touch than light touch, and want a sense of control over what is happening to their bodies. Teach the child to moisten and soap up her fingers and then use firm, circular motions—more like a massage than what we think of as face washing. She can develop a favored sequence, starting at, perhaps, the chin, doing the left cheek, then the right cheek, then the forehead. If the child is too young or otherwise unable to wash her own face, the parent can do it, talking the child through the sequence steps.

• Some people prefer a washcloth or buffing pad rather than fingertips. Experiment to find the optimal texture.

• Rinsing by splashing the face with water while keeping eyes tightly shut is often hard for kids to tolerate. First, experiment with temperature; a child might prefer the water slightly cooler or warmer than what the parent thinks is the right temperature. It may help to count down to "clean off," usually 6 to 10 good splashes of water. A child may prefer using a wet washcloth to carefully remove all facial cleanser while looking in the mirror.

Bathing and Showering

Some kids and adults, including those with tactile defensiveness, absolutely adore taking baths. The even, hydrostatic pressure envelops and soothes the body, providing the sustained tactile input many people crave. Water—via bathtub, shower, pool, lake, or other source—can be an important state changer, literally washing away bad feelings, worries, upsets, and other brain monsters. Water can help bring the person to that ideal state of calm alertness in the morning as well as lower arousal at the end of the day, enabling the person to drift off to sleep.

Yet for some, bathing and showering is not so easy. Feeling ungrounded while floating around in a bathtub or insecure when standing with eyes closed in the shower can be frightening for someone with poor body awareness, vestibular difficulties, or low muscle tone. A child may object to the sound of water against the tub or shower floor, the lighting, and the smell and texture of shampoo and conditioner, body wash, and other bathing products. The following are some ways to help.

Postural support. Parents should always provide a nonskid bathmat during showers and baths to avoid slips and falls. They can also install strategically placed grab bars so the person can hold onto something when he closes his eyes. Attaching an unbreakable mirror at eye level may help the individual to position herself in space when her eyes are open, and also help clue her in on when she needs to close her eyes.

Young children petrified by the expanse of the bathtub may do well in a smaller space like a bucket or large sink. It's easy to find baby and toddler bath seats with straps for very young children in stores that sell baby items. If an older child, teen, or even adult feels unmoored or is at risk for falling when he closes his eyes, he can sit on a bath chair, found in a medical supply or hardware store. If more support is needed for an older child, teen, or young adult, the Leckey Advance Bath Chair provides maximum support and stability for bathing. It is found in some therapy catalogs and online at places like www.adaptivemall.com.

Temperature. Kids with sensory issues may perceive hot and cold differently. Allow for exploration of cooler to warmer water to find ideal temperature within a safety zone. Parents can set a maximum temperature on the water heater and, to further avoid scalding, they can install the H2OT STOP antiscald shower head, tub spout, or hand shower from places like baby supply, home furnishing, or hardware stores. When hot water reaches an unsafe temperature, the H2OT STOP reduces water flow to a trickle to avoid scalding and restarts once the water cools down.

The child may also be more comfortable in the tub or shower if the parent warms up the room and surfaces by running warm water for a few minutes before having the child step in. Towels can also be preheated in the dryer before using.

Sensory Input. For many kids, bath time is a great time for sensory stimulation and exploration. Parents can provide tub toys such as tub paints, tub crayons, water whistles, squirt toys, and so on. Like everything else sensory, it takes some trial and error. One child might be afraid of bubbles and prefer plain water baths. Another may need those bubbles to maintain interest. Don't assume that soft is always best. In the tub or shower, a child might like a soft soapy massage or prefer a rigorous scrub-down with a loofah or a nylon net sponge. Experiment with whether the child reacts best by drying off with a fluffy soft towel or a towel with a stiffer texture.

Keep a bottle of water nearby in case the child gets thirsty. You don't want him drinking tub water if it is soapy and if there is any possibility that an older porcelain tub is releasing lead into the water. Parents can get a lead test kit from a hardware store.

When possible, children should pick out the products they like best. Fragrance-free, 100 percent organic shampoos, conditioners, soap, and bubble bath from companies like the Honest Co. (honest.com) are safest and best tolerated by sensitive people who cannot tolerate synthetic perfumes, dyes, and chemicals. Of course, some kids prefer intensely scented products such as Herbal Essences shampoo.

Shampooing and Rinsing. Many children enjoy baths and showers, but hate hair washing because they dislike the sensation of water sprinkled on the face and scalp. They also may dislike keeping their eyes squeezed shut and of course getting soap or water in the eyes. Once the child discovers a favorite shampoo and conditioner (combined rather than separate products may be best since this cuts the down on steps), parents can also:

- Desensitize the head first by gently but firmly massaging the scalp, ears, neck, and even the face. They can try a vibrating hairbrush (available from Amazon.com and many therapy catalogs). An oral vibrator on the cheeks, jaws, and lips may also be helpful.
- Consider whether the child would benefit from and tolerate noise-reducing or swimming earplugs (available at the drugstore or earplugstore.com).
- Pour water from a cup or a bucket for more even pressure while rinsing. Let the child dump the water out if possible. In either case, count down to the pouring so the child feels some predictability.
- A child might also be amenable to using a handheld shower head even if sitting in the tub. Explore different settings such as slow versus fast massaging pulse.
- The child can cover her eyes with a washcloth during shampooing and while rinsing off.
- A bath visor such as the Lil Rinser or Sassy Suds from stores or Diapers.com help keep water and shampoo out of eyes.
- Teach the child to shampoo her own hair as early as possible to encourage a sense of control and mastery.
- If absolutely necessary, use no-rinse shampoos such as TRESemmé Fresh Start Waterless Foam Shampoo, KMS Dry Shampoo, or other products available in many drugstores and online beauty supply sites.
- Play music in the shower or tub with a Shower-Tunes Water-Resistant Radio or Wet Tunes Shower Radio from Brookstone or

---

Disinfect Safely

Avoid products containing triclosan, an antibacterial/antimicrobial chemical originally developed as a pesticide. It's found in popular hand sanitizers, soaps, toothpaste, deodorant, and other hygiene products as well as in household products such as kitchen cutting boards. Laboratory studies prove this chemical interferes with skeletal and heart muscle function, hormonal regulation, and antibiotic resistance, although the Food and Drug Administration states that it doesn't have enough evidence about effects on humans for an outright ban. Visit the FDA Web site for more information and updates.

Some great alternatives for disinfecting include:

• CleanWell Foaming Hand Sanitizer, All-Natural Hand Sanitizing Wipes, and All-Natural, and Antibacterial Foaming Hand Soap, also available in industrial dispensers for schools, day care facilities, offices, and elsewhere
• The Honest Co.'s Honest Hand Sanitizer, Honest Wipes, and Honest Hand Soap
• Seventh Generation Purifying Handwash and disinfecting cleaning products
• BabyGanics Fine and Handy foaming hand soap and Germinator Hand Sanitizer

All are available online (search by product name) and in some retail stores such as Whole Foods and Bed Bath & Beyond.

---

online, experimenting with whether playing music is soothing or overstimulating. Cut a sponge or bar of soap into the shape of a microphone for some rock star action.

Hair Brushing and Haircutting

Hair brushing can be very hard for kids with a sensitive scalp, typically girls with longer hair that snarls easily. Haircuts present additional challenges, including the sound of scissors or a barber's hair buzzer, the smell of hair chemicals in a salon, and more. Here are some suggestions:

• Prior to brushing or a haircut, a parent can desensitize a child's scalp with a firm massage or pressing downward and inward with hands cradling the top of the head. Again, a vibrating hairbrush can be helpful.
• The child can wear a weighted vest, lap pad, or blanket if that's helpful.
• Encourage a positive experience by having the child listen to favorite music or watch a video.

- A good quality leave-in hair conditioner or spray-on detangling product smooths down the hair cuticle and reduces hair knotting. Ones to try include Jason Natural Products Kids Only Detangling Conditioner, Rainbow Research's Unscented Detangling Conditioner, and L'Oréal's Tangle Tamer.

- To avoid yanking hair, detangle with fingers first, then brush or comb starting with the hair ends while holding clumps of hair near the scalp.

- Try a special brush or comb such as the Knot Genie Hair Detangling Brush, Tangle Teezer Detangling brush, Goody Ouchless Comfort Gel Brush, or Detangling Comb.

At the barbershop or hair salon:

- If the child is prone to hair knots, consider cutting hair shorter or at least thinning thick hair. Be cautious with keratin hair treatments that relax curly hair as some lower-quality formulas contain a small amount of formaldehyde. Brazilian Blowouts should absolutely be avoided due to toxic formaldehyde fumes.

- Some kids do better with a soft, well-worn shirt from home and soft toweling around the neck than the barbershop or salon apron, especially if it has a scratchy Velcro closure behind the neck.

- Consider whether a child-oriented hair salon is overstimulating. Seats that look like cars, lots of balloons, a wall of videos, and lots of toys to buy can send some kids into overload, especially as someone approaches them with scissors.

- A smaller child may feel more secure sitting in a parent's lap than high up in a barber's chair.

- Say "trim, shorten, or style" instead of "cut" for kids who take words literally. "Cut" is a scary word!

- While a sensory seeker may be amused by the sound and vibration of the barber's hair buzzer, it may send a hypersensitive child into a meltdown. In such a case the barber can use scissors or at least have the child, wearing earplugs if need be, check out the buzzer more closely—observing it used on someone else, turning it on and off himself, and learning that it's weird but kind of cool.

- Hair procedures stink. If using an adult hair salon, schedule the appointment at a time when there will be no hair coloring, perming, or straightening being done.

• Finally, consider trimming the child's hair at home. You might even cut it while she is sleeping.

Sun Protection

Exposure to strong sunlight may be difficult for the sensitive child whose eyes and skin can hurt when light is too bright or glaring. Here are some suggestions:

• While parents usually won't send a child out in the sun for hours without sunblock, they may need a reminder to protect the child's eyes from sun too. Kids, teens, and adults should wear optical-quality sunglasses with anti-glare UV coating. Tint color is best left to personal preference, though neutral gray is often most acceptable since it doesn't significantly alter colors. While it seems logical to opt for super-dark shades, really dark lenses make pupils dilate, letting in even more light. Parents can ask an optometrist for the best lenses, even if nonprescription. Teens may especially enjoy the cool factor of wearing sunglasses. Younger and athletic kids can wear an added neoprene strap if needed. A hat or visor with a wide brim offers some additional eye protection.

• At the beach or lake, use an umbrella or tent to create shade and shelter.

• Some kids really dislike the way sunblock feels when applied. The parent can use firm massage-like strokes to apply sunscreen lotion rather than a tickly light touch.

• Experiment with lotions and spray-on sunscreens to find the most acceptable formulation, keeping in mind that although sprays may be more sensory friendly (or not), there is less guarantee that all areas will get coverage. With the sprays, be sure the child does not accidentally breathe any in by having her cover her mouth with a hand or towel. When applying lotion, use a golf ball–size amount and reapply every hour or so, even if it says it is waterproof.

• The child may be more able to tolerate sunscreen and sand if the parents does therapeutic brushing first, as shown by an occupational therapist.

• We're all so careful to use sunblock to protect against harmful UV rays that it comes as a surprise to learn that many of the chemicals in the sunblock are quite harmful themselves. Look for a formulation that is labeled broad-spectrum protection, and try to avoid oxy-benzone.You can find the safest sunblocks and sunscreens on the Environmental Working Group (EWG) Web site (see box below).

- Put sunscreen on the child before going to the beach or lake to give it time to dry and attract less sand and dirt. Plus it may be easier to tolerate at home where there is less conflicting sensory input.

- Kids can wear water shoes when walking on hot sand. Sand really can be too hot for sensitive young skin.

Hooray for EWG!

All kids (and adults) should avoid toxic chemicals whenever possible. This is particularly true for people with sensory challenges whose bodies tend to be extra-sensitive and susceptible to toxins. The EWG Web site (ewg.org) is a great source of reliable information and safety ratings for consumer products such as cosmetics, suntan lotion, household cleansers, and more. EWG is perhaps most famous for its Shopper's Guide to Pesticides in Produce, including the "dirty dozen" fruits and veggies that you should be sure to buy organic to reduce serious pesticide exposure.

Nail Clipping and Grooming

The fingertips and toes have so many nerve endings that it's no wonder many kids hate having their nails clipped. Some tricks:

- As with haircutting, use words such as "trim, shorten, file down" instead of "cut" for concrete thinkers.

- Teach parents to desensitize the skin by massaging the child's hands and giving extra input to the fingertips by gently compressing each nail between the thumb and index finger.

- Let the child wear a weighted vest, lap pad, or blanket and distract him with a video or music.

- Clip nails after bathing or showering when they are softer. This is also when you will want to remove any dirt under the nails. Don't dig too deeply, as it can be very painful. Better to soak it out in a bowl full of soapy water than dig it out.

- Use an emery board to gently file down nails instead of a clipper. Teach sensitive kids how to file down their own nails as young as possible so they can take control of their experiences.

- Some girls will tolerate nail grooming better if it's done at the beauty salon or manicure shop.
- If your child wears nail polish, keep in mind that most polishes contain toxic chemicals. The big three are formaldehyde (preservative, sterilizer, and embalming fluid), dibutyl phthalate (flexibility in plastics), and toluene (polish smoother and thinner known to affect the nervous system). Some safer polishes are made by OPI, Wet N Wild, and Sally Hansen, per the EWG.
- Some kids do best if you trim their nails while they are sleeping.

Brushing Teeth

Ask a friend or colleague to brush your teeth and you'll readily see how incredibly invasive tooth brushing really is. It's no wonder sticking a foreign object in your child's mouth can be perceived as uncomfortable, weird, or downright scary. Add in tactile issues with the lips, tongue, gums, and cheeks and you can see how tooth brushing and going to the dentist become battlegrounds for some families. Here are some tips for parents:

- Allow some control over tools, tastes, and texture. Let the child pick out a soft, child-size toothbrush in a favorite color with, perhaps, her beloved Hello Kitty or Elmo. Let her try out several flavors of toothpaste. The child who can't stand mint might accept a chocolate- or berry-flavored toothpaste. Kids and even adults with sensory issues may react negatively to the foam that forms as they brush. Nonfoaming toothpastes include Orajel Toddler Very Berry Training Toothpaste, Cha Cha Chocolate Toothpaste, and Tom's of Maine Orange-Mango Toothpaste.
- Many children and adults prefer using vibrating toothbrushes and do a more thorough job with them. Spin brushes are a decent, less costly alternative.
- Kids love timers and songs. The ideal brushing time is 2 minutes. Parents can set a timer, play a 2-minute song, or use an app such as the free Tooth Brushing Timer (iPad app). Some vibrating toothbrush models come with a digital monitor that shows how much time is left.

- Develop a predictable routine for brushing and provide a numbered picture chart if need be. For example, the child can always start with the top teeth, working from left to right, and then going to the bottom teeth from left to right. This will help your child to sequence this tricky task and predict when and where he will feel the brush in his mouth.

- Provide a model by brushing your teeth at the same time to make it a fun, shared experience.

Other ideas to promote oral-motor sensory comfort:

- Work on mouth skills such as sucking liquids through straws and water bottles with sports nozzle tops; chewing and crunching on foods such as chewing gum, pretzels, and carrot sticks; biting and pulling on licorice strings and fruit roll-ups; and licking lollipops and fruit pops.

- Increase mouth awareness and normalize sensitivity level (so the mouth is neither over- nor undersensitive). For younger kids, parents can massage gums. A therapist may show parents or older children how to use an oral vibrator.

- Make funny noises (blow raspberries, noisy kisses, pops, clicks) and make funny faces at each other.

- Play tongue taste games. Sweet is detected by taste receptors at the front of the tongue, salty at the sides of the tongue tip, sour and spicy on the middle sides, and bitter and smoky toward back of the tongue.

Loose Teeth

Losing teeth can be especially momentous for a child with oral defensiveness who may be equally freaked out by having a loose or dangling tooth and by the notion of having it pulled out. If the child can tolerate cold, have her suck on an ice pop to numb the area if the tooth needs yanking.

There are loads of books on this subject that you can read together such as *My Wobbly Tooth Must Not Ever Never Fall Out* by Lauren Child. Many parents have posted videos of their child's first loose tooth on YouTube. Parents can find a video with a child of the same approximate age as their own and watch it together, with the parent previewing it to make sure it is suitable.

Toileting

Learning to use the toilet can be a snap for the child who does not like to be messy. Some virtually toilet train themselves. Others need help, especially if they have difficulty sensing when their bowel or bladder is full, don't detect when they are messy, or actually enjoy that wet or poopy feeling.

Remember that getting to the toilet in time requires neurological maturity and interoceptive development (monitoring bowel and bladder sensations) and that kids reach the toilet-ready state at different times, quite often later for a child hitting other developmental milestones late too. Several excellent books on this topic are available, including *Toilet Training for Individuals With Autism or Other Developmental Issues* by Maria Wheeler.

Here are a few sensory suggestions for when the child shows signs of being ready to toilet train:

- Underwear briefs that fit snugly over the bladder may interfere with processing the sensation of a full bladder. Opt for looser boxer-style underwear available for both boys and girls.

- If a child has trouble feeling when he is messy, take him to the toilet at regular intervals. Neutrally state whether he or she is dry or messy and neutrally narrate what is going on: either that the child is dry so you'll visit the bathroom again later or oops, the child has peed or pooped on himself instead of in the toilet but you'll try to get to the bathroom in time next time.

- Provide the best sitting experience. While one small child might appreciate sitting on a little plastic potty on the floor, another might be happier on the big-kid toilet with a pull-down toilet adapter seat or a cute seat insert decorated with a favorite character such as Winnie the Pooh. In either case, make sure the child has support under her feet, with feet flat on the floor or on a footstool. This is especially important for a child who has poor muscle tone and postural control.

Getting Dressed

Many children, teens, and adults have strong likes and dislikes when it comes to clothing due to tactile sensitivities and sometimes visual, smell, and other sensitivities. Parents may have first noticed that their baby has a meltdown whenever his diaper is changed. This may be due to abrupt changes in head and body position as he is placed on a changing table, the way he is physically handled by his caregiver, or the feeling of the powder, lotion, or diaper itself.

Later, there may be particular textures, seams, patterns, colors, and styles the child just can't stand. In some cases, it may take a very long time until she finds something that feels just right to wear. A child may insist on wearing just one or two particular T-shirts. Another may be willing to wear only blue clothing. Getting kids dressed in the morning can become a nightmare for parents and children, putting everyone in a bad mood before school and work.

A student who is aware of his sock seams pressing against his toes and his shirt cuffs chafing against his wrists all day long may struggle to focus on classwork. In the middle of a snowstorm, a child may be absolutely unable to tolerate wearing a hat, gloves, and winter boots. In summer, a child may insist on long sleeves and long pants. A teenager may be embarrassed by his "dorky" sweatpants, unable to wear the blue jeans every cool kid in school wears because they make him feel squeezed, rubbed raw, and claustrophobic. A girl who can't tolerate wearing a frilly party dress like her girlfriends because it tickles her too much may feel like an outsider.

Many parents become understandably frustrated by catering to their child's clothing preferences. In-laws and others may be particularly unkind here, blaming the mom or dad for indulging the child in this "silliness." While pickiness about clothing may well have a behavioral aspect, it's helpful to remind parents that children with sensory issues often have problems in this area due to their neurological differences. And like so many other sensory issues, it will get better in time with help from an OT who can decrease the child's tactile sensitivity while reasonably accommodating the special needs.

Predictability can help. Have the child pick out what he will wear the night before. If the child thrives on visual schedules such as calendars and meal menus, create a clothing schedule. If a parent finds an acceptable T-shirt, buy several. If a child has a color preference, allow him to pick clothing in that color. Try building in some variety by adding stripes, polka dots, or other patterns that include additional colors. Here are more clothing strategies:

- Wash new clothes multiple times in hot water to remove the sizing that can make clothing stiff and uncomfortable. This will also help remove any residual pesticide from clothing shipped from overseas. Consider buying "preconditioned" clothing from a consignment or thrift shop.

- If the child is sensitive to chemicals and dyes, buy organic fabrics only, which tend to be softer and cozier anyway.

- Avoid clothing treated with fire-retardant chemicals, which studies have begun to show are toxic and hormone disrupting.

- Avoid fabric softener because it contains small amounts of potentially dangerous chemicals that can trigger itchy skin and respiratory problems. Stay on the safe side and go green as much as possible with all personal and household products.

- Parents can take the child shopping during off hours or shop together online. This will let the child feel more in control of what happens to his body.

- Eliminate or avoid clothing irritants such as tags, labels, scratchy threads, elastic cuffs, elastic ankles, and waistbands, tight collars and turtlenecks, and appliqués. Teach parents to run fingers along sewn sections to feel for scratchiness, lumps, and bumps. If clothing irritants cannot be avoided (the child has to wear a certain uniform or adores a shirt that actually bothers her), parents can cover the offending seam, tab, or whatever with Undercover Tape (from mimilounge.com and some retailers). It's not a permanent solution, but it will last for multiple washings. Stick-on moleskin may also work, though it can leave a sticky residue on clothing.

- Work with an occupational therapist to learn tactile desensitization techniques such as deep pressure and joint compression prior to dressing.

- Exfoliate flaky, dry skin and apply high-quality moisturizer to the child's body before dressing, especially in winter and dry climates.

- Some parents and therapists have good results with adding essential fatty acid supplements such as fish oil to the diet in terms of improved mood and behavior as well as reduced sensitivity to clothing.

- Explore different clothing options such as seamless socks or socks worn inside out; snug tights, leggings, and tops beneath regular clothing; clothing alternatives such as soft sweatpants or stretchy denim leggings instead of blue jeans.

There are now several companies that specialize in sensory-friendly clothing, including these:

- EZ Socks (ezsocks.com): These socks for kids and adults have easy-to-grip pull loops that make it easier for kids to learn to put on their socks as well as for teens and adults with limited hand dexterity and coordination, poor mobility, and more.

- Fun and Function (funandfunction.com): A cute assortment of short and long-sleeved Sens-ational Hug shirts provides calming, gentle compression that can be worn alone or under clothing.

- Hanna Andersson (hannaandersson.com): High-quality, soft clothing and undergarments for babies, children, and women. Several styles of sensory-friendly underwear for boys and girls do not have irritating gathered waistbands.

- SmartKnit Kids (smartknitkids.com): Seamless knit socks that wick away moisture for kids, teens, and adults plus seamless knit underwear for boys and girls, plus seamless "bralettes" and compression tank tops. Also has seamless socks for kids who wear AFO and KAFO orthotics.

- Soft Clothing (softclothing.net): Soft, tagless tops, bottoms (including faux denim pants), dresses, blazers, and coats for boys and girls. Very soft, seamless polyester-spandex socks. Seamless, organic cotton underwear for boys and girls.

- Teres Kids (tereskids.com): 100 percent American organic cotton, tag-free clothing line with seams cleverly sewn flat on the outside, including short- and long-sleeve shirts, dresses, leggings, and pants for boys and girls.

Parents can increasingly find sensory-friendly clothing in stores, including Hanes seamless, tagless underwear and soft girls' clothing by Velvet, Splendid, and others. Some kids and teens like the snug compression of UnderArmour sports clothing, Lycra bicycle clothing, control-top tights, and so on.

Mealtime

Too many of today's families are overscheduled and rushed. Between long hours for working parents, multiple after-school activities, and more homework than ever, there just never seems to be enough time. This gets even harder when soccer practice runs late for one child, another child has an evening tutoring session, and one parent has to work overtime. Kids and parents wind up eating in shifts, so everyone gets shortchanged.

Constant rushing and haphazard eating schedules are especially hard on supersensitive kids, who tend to be creatures of habit. Try to serve meals at the same time every day to establish a mealtime routine and encourage regular hunger-satiety cycles. If at all possible, have everyone in the family sit down together for meals—at least a few nights a week. It may seem old fashioned and outmoded to some super-busy parents, but the dinner table is where families have traditionally socialized and where children learn table manners and eating habits.

Here are some strategies to make sitting down for meals easier:

Seating Considerations

Some parents complain that their child will not remain seated at the table during meals or that the child slouches down in the seat, falls off the chair, or pushes against other people with their feet, or kicks others under the table. These behaviors can be quite annoying and downright disruptive when the family is trying to have a nice meal together.

Sitting at a table can be very difficult for the SPD child. If he has low core muscle tone, his muscles can't fight the force of gravity for long. Even if he initially sits with an upright posture, he usually can't sustain it and soon enough will start sinking like a wet noodle, slouching into a spinal C-curve with a posteriorly tilted pelvis and often straightened legs. He may slide right out of his chair or simply sit in this "bad attitude" posture, which also restricts breathing, swallowing, and visual attention. To compensate, he may drape his body over the table, prop his elbows on the table to support his upper body and head, or move frequently to keep his trunk muscles active. A child with poor body awareness who does not properly perceive where her body parts are may also be struggling to sit upright and still as expected. To increase proprioceptive input into her legs and trunk, she may push against a chair leg, sibling, or parent with her feet. The child who is overaroused may have great difficulty reaching a calm, organized state and remain still and seated, instead seeking out movement input by wiggling, fidgeting, and getting out of the seat.

Seating Strategies for Mealtimes and Other Tabletop Activities

- Prior to sitting down, engage the child in sensory activities that are calming and organizing. These might include jumping on a mini-trampoline, doing jumping jacks, climbing a few flights of stairs, using an oral vibrator, bouncing while sitting on a therapy ball, or just some quiet time to regroup before eating.

- Make sure the chair and table are the right size. When a child has low muscle tone, poor strength, or poor body awareness, it is especially important to have a chair and table that are appropriate to his body proportions. When seated at a table, the child's arms should slope down to the tabletop (as opposed to having to reach up), and forearms should be able to rest comfortably on the tabletop; the hips should be at a more or less 90-degree angle (right angle) on the seat; knees should also be at an approximate 90-degree angle; and feet should reach the floor in a flat, relaxed position.

- The right chair can make an enormous difference. Rather than having a small child sit in an adult chair with a booster seat, parents should seriously consider special seating such as the Tripp Trapp Chair (online or at many children's furniture departments). This chair grows along with the child so that he's always at the right height with a footrest. Rifton chairs (Rifton.com) have armrests plus optional foot supports and leg positioners that can enable the child with both low and high muscle tone to sit comfortably for longer periods. Ergonomic desk chairs for kids such as the DuoRest

Student Desk Chair provide nice back support with optional armrests and footrests that can help an older child sit and do homework
for long periods more comfortably. Other seating adaptations can
easily be found online on sites such as adaptivemall.com.

• The feet always form the base of support for the rest of the body. If
the child's feet cannot reach the floor, as is often the case when sitting on adult-sized furniture, a footrest needs to be added such as:

– Right size box with nonskid matting beneath it.

– Footstool with a rubberized base such as those from Ikea or
Baby Bjorn.

– A Movin' Step, an inflatable foot cushion available in therapy and
exercise catalogs, an especially nice choice for a child who is
always pushing against something or someone, as he can push
into the foot cushion to get the input he craves without bothering anyone.

– Kickers may be satisfied and focused if they are able to push
against some Theraband or Lycra tied across the front chair legs,
provided the child is not at risk for tripping on it.

– Just Foam premade foam blocks (in therapy catalogs or make
them yourself out of dense foam).

– Yoga blocks.

• The pelvis and buttocks should be in a neutral position to promote
an erect spine with ribcage neither caved in or jutting out. A seat
cushion and possibly back support can be added to promote postural alignment and increase seating comfort, such as these:

– Disc 'O' Sit cushion, Swiss Disc, and other round inflatable seat
cushions provide "dynamic sitting" that lets kids wiggle, that is,
actively move trunk and hip muscles while remaining seated.

– A Movin' Sit cushion is a wedge-shaped inflatable cushion. With
the wide edge toward the back of the chair, when lightly inflated,
this cushion helps move a posteriorly tilted pelvis (slouched)
into a more neutral, upright position and provides an active seating surface that keeps muscles working.

– Memory Foam seat cushions and other molded seat cushions.

– Meditation cushions and semi-firm pillows.

– As adult seats are generally too deep for a child to get any back
support without slumping, parents can add support by building

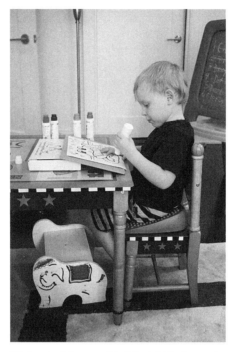

Richard sitting on his Movin' Sit Jr. cushion. *Photo courtesy of author*

up the back of the seat. A semi-firm pillow, rolled towels, or add-on cushions such as a strap-on back cushion or lumbar support can work well.

• Stabilizing the forearms on a tabletop promotes better upper body stability and hand use. The child should never have to hike up her shoulders or lift her arms significantly to reach for something on the table. A seat cushion can be added to raise the child up with foot support added if necessary.

• If the child has gravitational insecurity, she may feel lost in space and unanchored sitting so high up in an adult chair. This child would likely benefit from:

– Being seated next to a wall

– Sitting in a chair with arms, possibly with pillows or rolled towels on either side so she feels supported

– Sitting in a chair with a safety belt such as the Tripp Trap

– Having foot support

• Provide sensory tools to help kids stay seated. For some kids, a weighted wearable such as a lap pad, vest, or shoulder wrap add enough calming proprioceptive input to keep them seated. An oral comfort tool such as a Chewy Tube or Kids Companion or hand fidget such as a squeeze ball or Rubik's cube can also help an antsy child stay put with the family even when he's not eating. A visual such as the Time Timer will help fidgety kids understand how long they are being asked to sit for (see Chapter 7).

Utensils and Dishware

Children may be sensitive to the type of utensil used in terms of shape, size, and feel on the handle or the mouthing surface. Others may have difficulty physically grasping a fork, knife or spoon. Fortunately, a wide variety of eating utensils is available:

• For children who cannot tolerate metal in their mouths, or who react badly to the sound of metal on a plate, parents can offer plastic utensils and plates, watching out for scratchy edges. Even better in terms of avoiding plastics, parents can check out the Bambu Kids line of ecologically sustainable bamboo forks, spoons, knives, and plates (Bambuhome.com). Bambu Home also offers fun sporks (a combined fork and spoon) that kids may enjoy.

• Some kids may prefer eating with wood or lacquer chopsticks or Zoo Sticks or Fish Sticks, fun tongs available in many toy stores and therapy catalogs.

• Look for spoons that are not too wide for the child's mouth. A deeper spoon bowl makes it easier for a child to scoop up food without it falling off the side. Forks with tines that actually spear food rather than rounded tips are much more effective, safety permitting. If grasp is a problem, look for rounded and textured handles that make holding on easier. Gripables cutlery (from thepencilgrip.com, therapro.com, and others online) is ergonomically designed with a metal eating surface and a comfortable padded handle for easy grasp and use. Sassy makes some cute textured plastic ware. Evo.OTware (available from evopen.com) is especially easy to use for teens and adults with grasp difficulties due to arthritis, cerebral palsy, hemiplegia, and other physical impairments.

• Weighted utensils from therapy catalogs give extra proprioceptive input that can help some hands. KEatlery weighted utensils look like a normal utensil, which may be ideal for a teen or young adult, while the pediatric and adult weighted or coated utensils have large, weighted handles added on. Therapro (therapro.com) has a nice selection of weighted utensils.

• Kids can get frustrated when they are trying to scoop up food and the dish is sliding around. Use a nonskid placemat or Dycem. Look for a bowl with a suction cup base and a plate with an edge so food doesn't just slide off (sites such as therapro.com). Make sure the bowl or plate you serve food in doesn't have a notched ridge that makes it hard to get the food up.

• Using a funny straw can make drinking any liquid more fun. You can add soothing sensory input by having kids drink thicker liquids such as liquid yogurt and smoothies through a straw.

• Many alternative cups are available that can make drinking easier, such as the Mr. Juice Bear and Nosey Cup, which has a cutout on the nondrinking side so it can be tilted without banging into the nose. Again, Therapro has a great selection of cups and straws.

• If the child has trouble using utensils and cups, consult with an OT. There are many adapted utensils, dishes, and cups in therapy catalogs.

Eating Environments

Children who are sensitive to environmental factors such as lighting, ventilation, smells, and noise may be poor eaters only in certain environments.

At Home. Parents can take steps to ensure that the eating area is sensory friendly for the child. Replace fluorescent lighting if possible, and if not, use natural lighting, a lamp with full-spectrum or incandescent bulbs, or a warm white LED lamp. Seat the child away from odor sources including cooking smells, garbage, and dirty diapers. Watching TV or a video during mealtimes is not advised, although some parents find it's the only way to get their child to eat. Listening to favorite music is preferable.

At School. Lunch can be an unsavory time for students with sensory issues due to embarrassing picky eating issues plus smell, auditory sensitivity, and other issues if they eat in a school cafeteria. Please see Chapter 7 for school lunch strategies.

In Restaurants. Eating out presents a host of additional challenges for the sensitive child, including unfamiliar foods and smells, the clatter of a commercial kitchen, the noise of other customers and piped-in music, different seating, linens, tableware, and so much more.

For sensory seekers, the novelty of eating out can be so enticing that they are actually willing to try something new even if they are picky eaters. A child may be so excited about finally getting to go to the chain restaurant she has seen in TV commercials that she is actually willing to eat her adored coconut shrimp even if it does have parsley or is spicier than she is accustomed to.

Restaurants can be very hard for more aversive eaters. A parent may become frustrated when the family goes to a restaurant and orders the hamburger and fries the child loves at the local diner only to find that the child won't eat it because the hamburger doesn't taste exactly the same and the fries aren't crinkle-cut. It may well be that the overall noise level or lighting makes eating even familiar foods too difficult.

Here are suggestions for a parent who knows that eating out is likely to be problematic:

- Bring along food that the child can tolerate, even if it is a protein bar or sandwich. The waiter will forgive the parent more readily for doing this than if the child has a complete meltdown at the table.

- Bring along an age-appropriate busy bag. For a young child this may include crayons and a notepad, a picture book, play dough, and a stuffed toy. An older child may be able to keep behavior organized by drawing, playing a handheld video game, or listening to music over headphones. Yes, it's not so social, but it is better than having a meltdown in the middle of a restaurant.

- If necessary, bring your own utensils and seating adaptations. The child who manages to eat well using a spoon with a built-up handle should have it with him. As most restaurant chairs are the wrong size for kids, bring along any seating adaptation such as an inflatable seat cushion or footrest that the child is accustomed to using.

• There is a big difference between restaurants in terms of sensory challenge. If possible, prescreen the restaurant for how closely positioned the tables are, noise level including both people and music, downcast lighting, and so on. Ask for a table in the quietest spot possible, and do not hesitate to ask the manager to lower the music.

Food Issues

Nourishing a child is one of the most basic parental responsibilities. Eating a limited number of foods and asking for the same foods over and over can be annoying, but it's actually developmentally typical for young children. In one study, between the ages of 4 and 24 months, the percentage of children identified as picky eaters by their caregivers increased from 19 percent to 50 percent (Caruth, Ziegler, Gordon, & Barr, 2004).

Like so many things, difficulties with feeding run on a spectrum, from picky eaters to problem eaters to virtual noneaters. Picky eaters tend to limit their food repertoire to 25–35 different foods. Although parents may get impatient with catering to their demands, these children eat enough calories daily to maintain a healthy weight and thrive. They may be rigid about what they are willing to eat. A child may insist on exactly the same brand of macaroni and cheese cooked exactly the same way and served in a certain bowl at a particular temperature. It takes a lot of time, patience, and repeated food trials to get such a child to try a new food, which she may well enjoy once she accepts a tiny nibble. For these kids, "try it, you'll like it" actually works if a parent introduces a new food several times.

Children with medical issues and feeding problems are another story altogether. These are children who, for physical reasons such as severe gastroesophageal reflux disease, celiac disease, Hirschsprung's disease, or other conditions, struggle or fail to thrive because they are unable to eat enough to gain adequate calories and nutrients from what they ingest orally.

Kids with SPD usually fall somewhere in the middle of this spectrum. Food repertoires tend to be extremely limited, often encompassing less than 20 acceptable foods. Unlike the child with a psychiatric eating disorder, these children are willing to eat, but only those foods that their senses are able to tolerate. There are generally no worries about weight gain or body dysmorphic features, although they may be on the lower end of percentiles for height and weight because of their limited diets.

Tactile hypersensitivity on the lips, tongue, roof of mouth, inside cheeks, and throat may make it seem unbearable to eat foods that have certain textures—most often lumpy, slippery, dry and crumbly, or combined textures such as yogurt mixed with granola.

Kids with oral tactile undersensitivity may pocket food around their cheeks and gums without noticing. To compensate, they may stuff their mouths in order to feel that something's in there and then be at risk for choking. They may seek out foods that have intense flavors, adding hot sauce to scrambled eggs and slathering spicy mustard onto barbecued chicken.

Some are particular about food aromas and flavors and may eat only foods that are bland, sweet, or salty. Some kids will eat foods only at a certain temperature. Another child may eat a balanced meal if food is served slightly chilled, including meats and vegetables. Yet another child will eat only if food is served lukewarm or steaming hot. These kinds of eating demands can make parents feel like short-order cooks. Harried and frustrated ones.

Other kids object to the way food looks or when items touch each other on a plate. They may become very rigid about eating just one brand of cereal in one special bowl with just one particular spoon.

Some problem feeders lack strength and stability in the lips, tongue, and jaw early on for nursing and later on when learning to eat solid foods. Jaw weakness makes eating crunchy and chewy foods difficult while tongue weakness makes it hard to form the round food mass called a bolus needed to swallow. High or low muscle tone in the mouth can also interfere with feeding. If the child has a hyperactive gag reflex, he'll avoid eating food that is likely to make him gag. If he has success with a particular food, he may self-limit to that one food.

At its most extreme, a child may throw up when an offending food is tasted, smelled, or just mentioned. In some cases, strong reactions to certain foods are due to zinc deficiency, notes nutritionist Kelly Dorfman (Dorfman, 2013). Dorfman says that children with low levels of zinc may perceive foods as unpleasant because their sense of smell and taste are altered.

Zinc deficiency may explain why so many children stick to a "white diet" consisting of pasta with butter, French fries, bread, pancakes, waffles, fish sticks, chicken nuggets, milk, cheese, and other pale, soft foods that have a mushy mouth feel. This diet lacks zinc and other important minerals. These foods are also heavy on gluten, the main protein in wheat, barley, and other grains, and casein, a protein found in cheese and other dairy products, which many kids with sensory problems actually do not tolerate well. Gluten or casein intolerance is different from an actual allergy. The theory is that these proteins trigger immune responses in some kids, resulting in a pleasurable high. Gluten and casein issues are worth exploring with a nutritionist or allergist if the child has gastrointestinal issues or frequent colds, sinus problems, or ear infections. A special diet free of artificial colorings and sweeteners called the Feingold Diet may also be worth looking into, especially for children with behavioral issues including hyperactivity (see feingold.org and gfcf.com).

Tips for Problem Eaters

Expanding food repertoires takes patience, creativity, and gentle insistence. One of the worst pieces of advice the parent of a truly picky eater, problem feeder, or noneater can receive is that if the child is hungry enough, he will eat. It's simply not true. When a child has a significantly limited food repertoire, he will go to bed hungry and develop nutritional deficiencies rather than eat something that he perceives as absolutely repulsive, scary, and dangerous. Parents most certainly should *not* withhold the few foods that are acceptable. If they take away that one brand of frozen fish sticks the child will eat for breakfast, lunch, and dinner, they're taking away the sole source of nutrition for the child, even if it is not the ideal one.

Many parents express frustration that the child won't try new foods. All too often that's because they try introducing several new foods at once, which then overwhelms the child. Parents should plan to identify just one food to slowly add to a child's diet, giving the child a choice between acceptable foods. For example, if the child likes salty foods, he might enjoy dehydrated, salted string beans, sold in the chips section at Trader Joe's and Whole Foods. He might then try lightly steamed and salted string beans.

Introducing a new food to a sensory-challenged child may take dozens of tries. Madison and her mom identified bananas as a food she would consider eating "in the future." Session 1: We made a collage of banana pictures. Real bananas were within sight. Sessions 2–4: she learned to slice bananas and fed them to her mother, in a playful, unpressured interaction. She smelled and felt the banana and observed her mother enjoying it. Sessions 5–8: She touched one banana slice to her lips before either feeding it to her mom or throwing it away. Sessions 9–12: She touched the banana slice with her tongue and threw it away. Sessions 13–14: She nibbled on the banana slice and then spit it onto a napkin. On the 15th session, she swallowed the nibble. Sessions 16–17: She ate one slice of banana. Session 18: She ate half a banana. Now she loves bananas and has selected sweet peas as a vegetable she will eat "when she is older."

While you do want to work on just one food at a time, don't give up introducing new foods. When it's dinnertime, go ahead and serve the child's favorite food but also make other food available on the table. However, if your child cannot bear strong food odors, such as brussel sprouts, she may be so nauseated that she will be unable to eat at all.

Here are a few additional ideas for families to try:

- Combine familiar foods with new ones, with full disclosure so the child doesn't feel tricked. A parent can add blueberries to pancakes or some fresh cheddar cheese to packaged macaroni and cheese. Dips work well too. If the child loves white potato fries smothered in ketchup, offer her ketchup for dipping sweet potato fries. If he loves cheese sauce, give him cheese sauce to dip a tree (broccoli) or a stick (string bean). Tahini, hummus, and duck sauce dips are all worth trying.

- Avoid filling up on empty calories like chips or sugary apple juice that offer virtually no nutrition. If the child constantly drinks juice, a parent can water it down slowly over the course of several weeks. Rather than giving a full bag of Veggie Booty which, like ketchup, does not count as a vegetable, serve a small bowlful.

- Avoid allowing a child to graze on food anywhere, anytime. Try to establish a feeding schedule to help establish hunger cycles. If the child must eat unexpectedly, he should be served sitting down. If the child gets up, the food should remain on the table.

- If the child is very resistant to any change, modify foods just slightly. Use large cookie cutters to make funny-shaped grilled cheese sandwiches and chop fresh berries into pudding.

- If the child thrives on predictability and having a sense of control, create a weekly written family menu with photos if needed.

- Provide nonfood "oral comforts" that help normalize mouth sensations. Some favorites include Chewy Tubes, Chew-Eaze, Dr. Bloom's Chewable Jewels, and KidCompanions Chewlery. You can find these in most therapy catalogs and online.

- Above all, teach families to avoid food battles. The family dinner is not therapy time. If the parent wishes to introduce a new food, do so earlier in the day when the child is not tired or stressed out. At the dinner table, parents should serve food they know the child will eat and focus on having pleasurable time together.

When to Refer to a Feeding Specialist

After ruling out any medical issues such as reflux or celiac disease, the family may need to work with a feeding specialist (typically an occupational therapist or speech language pathologist). Melanie Potock, a pediatric speech language pathologist, suggests parents consult with a feeding specialist if:

- The child is not following the typical growth curve for any of the following: height, weight, or head circumference.

- The child's diet is restricted to just certain foods that are unbalanced in terms of nutrition and/or variety such as only carbs, only protein, or just . . . pistachio nuts.

- The child is a messy eater and it is impacting social interactions or peer relationships.

- The child is anxious about trying new foods or eating in specific environments, such as the school cafeteria.

• The child's relationship with food is negatively impacting the family's relationship with food and thus, family behavior and family dynamics. (personal communication, October 7, 2012)

The feeding therapist will likely recommend oral desensitization and strengthening techniques and systematically work with the family to introduce new consistencies, textures, aromas, and tastes as well as to support the entire family in developing healthier food-related patterns.

You may also want to refer to a nutritionist who can correct any nutritional imbalances and boost the child's nervous system function. "Your brain is a mass of chemicals that rely totally on what is available for them to operate," says nutritionist Kelly Dorfman (personal communication, October 14, 2012). "Targeted nutrition therapy can benefit most cases. Getting a child into optimal nutritional shape means she will have the biochemical tools to thrive."

Parents may want to pay special attention to omega-3 fatty acids, especially EPA (eicosapentaenoic acid), which multiple studies show have a direct effect on brain and neuropsychiatric function. An increasing body of evidence shows that omega-3 fats may help improve symptoms of bipolar disorder, ADHD, anxiety, serotonin syndrome, Alzheimer's, schizophrenia, and other neuropsychiatric disorders (Dorfman, 2013; Stevens, Zentall, Abate, Kuczek, & Burgess, 1996; Stordy, 2000).

Parties, Holidays, and Other Group Gatherings

Birthday parties, family holidays and other group gatherings can be hard for sensitive kids. A parent who is accustomed to a child's likes and dislikes at home may be beside herself when she takes the child to a birthday party and watches him fall apart when everyone else sings "Happy Birthday" with glee. Getting together with relatives can highlight the child's sensory issues, as the sensory-based behaviors and compensations the parent takes for granted become a topic of discussion.

Just about every parent of a child who struggles with sensory issues has heard statements such as:

- Give him a week at my house, and I'll straighten him out.
- She just needs to get over it. Don't indulge her.
- Don't you ever just say no?

A parent may be understandably nervous about a child's behavior if he tends to act up or tune out in these situations. As much as possible, counsel parents to try to not to be self-conscious or apologetic about giving their child what his brain and body need. This is the perfect time to explain the child's sensory needs and how you are empowering her to overcome them. Praise and rewards are always appropriate if the child has behaved to the best of his or her ability. Parents are not spoiling kids when they celebrate success.

Before any party or group gathering, the parent can let the child know what to expect. If the gathering is in the child's own home, parents should review who will be coming and discuss something special about that person. You might mention that Aunt Rita just bought a new car or that Cousin Stella has a cat that likes to walk on a leash. If it's elsewhere, ask the host who will be there and what the plan is for the occasion.

Remind the child of social expectations. Indeed, he must greet each guest, but he does not have to kiss everyone. Instead, he can say hello and put his hand out for a handshake. Teach him about keeping most people at arm's length so he doesn't stand too close and become a space invader. Parents may need to help the child self-advocate around overbearing relatives that won't take no for an answer when it comes to unwelcome hugs and sloppy kisses.

Discuss an escape strategy if the child tends to become overloaded in these situations. Remind the child that if she starts feeling overloaded—perhaps scared, tired, frustrated, or even dizzy—she can approach the parent for help. Before the event, determine a spot where the child can go and what she can do if she begins to feel badly. It's much better for a child to take a short break from a gathering than to feel trapped in a situation that is veering toward sensory meltdown. If at home, let her know she can excuse herself to go to her room if she needs time to reorganize. If away from home, figure out a safe place for the child to retreat to such as a bedroom, a hallway, or elsewhere.

Kids can certainly bring along favorite activities and toys such as coloring supplies, a book, headphones with music, fidget tools, or whatever can be used without bothering others. Bring plenty for any other kids to enjoy and share easily, such an extra box of crayons, extra containers of Play-Doh, and so on. If the child loves using his iPad or other handheld device, he should be allowed to bring it along and use it at acceptable times. If it is used as an aid for communication, it should of course always be at hand.

It's never worth forcing kids into party clothing that makes them miserable. Itchy lace, elastic waistbands, and choking collars and ties may be absolutely intolerable. There are plenty of pretty dresses for girls that are also sensory friendly. A child who is very selective about clothing who needs to dress up can go ahead and wear that beloved Thomas the Tank Engine T-shirt beneath a dress shirt. Whatever special outfit the child wears, be sure to give it a test run a few times before the event, and have parents bring a change of clothing just in case.

Let the child know what foods are going to be served, keeping in mind that the food may look, smell, or taste differently when someone else makes it—and therefore not be acceptable to a picky eater. Parents shouldn't feel they need to force the child to eat something he finds "gross" just because it's the traditional holiday food. Parents should bring along something nutritious they know the child will eat rather than just loading up on high-carb side dishes. At the same time, a group gathering may be the time he'll finally try a new food, especially if an admired friend or relative enjoys it.

If parents feel judged or criticized about giving in to food issues, they can explain that food battles are counterproductive, and that while they are working on expanding the child's food repertoire, a holiday meal is certainly not the right time to work on it since the entire point is to enjoy being together.

Dentists, Doctors, and Other Professional Visits

Dentist

Going to the dentist presents a multitude of challenges on top of any oral sensitivity issues. Between the rubber gloves, harsh light, changes in head position as the chair tilts back, having a stranger's hands inside your mouth doing weird things you can't see, plus the sound of the drill, going to the dentist can be quite unpleasant, to put it mildly. There is a lot a parent can do to improve the experience for a child.

For starters, it's worth doing some research to find a dentist with child-friendly waiting and treatment rooms who is patient, compassionate, and willing to work with parents on making the visit as comfortable as possible. Have parents explain the child's sensory challenges and ask the dentist to begin the exam with his fingers or possibly a familiar toothbrush. To avoid surprises, ask the dentist to explain where he or she is about to touch the child, and to allow the child to see and touch dental tools before they are used.

Knowing what to expect can really help, though it's important to assess the amount of preparatory information that will be comforting versus the amount that will simply increase anxiety about the dentist. Have the child visit the dentist's office simply to check out the dentist, rooms, and equipment. Let the child observe a sibling or parent in the dentist chair since watching someone else getting his teeth checked and cleaned may reduce fears. The child can role-play going to the dentist with a therapist or parent, using a dental mirror, tongue depressors, gloves, and a bowl to spit in, being sure to take turns playing patient so the child has some control.

For a younger child, read a book about going to the dentist such as *The Berenstain Bears Visit the Dentist* or *Dora the Explorer's Show Me Your Smile! A Visit to the Dentist*. Some children may appreciate a simple, reassuring narrative about going to the dentist in the form of a Social Story, such as the real-life video of a child with autism (Aspergers Social Stories, 2012). Social Stories, developed by Carol Gray, use a specific style and format to explain a situation, skill, or concept to increase understanding of events and expectations (see thegraycenter.org).

Here are more ideas:

- If orally defensive, an occupational or speech therapist can teach the parent, older child, or teenager oral desensitization techniques using a vibrating teether or toothbrush, massaging gums with a Z-Vibe and textured tips, Den-Tips or Toothettes, or an oral vibrator such as Ellie the Elephant Jiggler.

- Ask the dentist to use gloves that are flavored, including cherry, grape, or bubble gum, from companies like Perfect Touch and Shamrock. If latex is a problem, your dentist can use pink or purple nonlatex gloves from Kimberly-Clark or Medline. They are all easily found on amazon.com. Use the same kind for preparatory role-playing.

- The child should be allowed to wear the weighted bib while in the chair for calming deep-pressure input, even when X-rays aren't being taken—or ask the dentist about having the child wear a weighted vest, weighted blanket, or weighted lap pad from home.

- The child can listen to music or wear noise-canceling ear protection while teeth are being cleaned or drilled.

- The child can wear sunglasses to protect eyes from the harsh lights. Ask the dentist to avoid shining the light directly into the eyes as much as possible.

- Some dentists have video screens for patients. If so, bring along a favorite video.

- The child can bring and use preferred toothpaste or mouth rinse.

- The child can hold a favorite hand fidget tool such as a squeeze ball, Tangle, beloved stuffed toy, or other security object.

- Moving into a reclining position and having the dentist chair raised and lowered can be really distressing for kids with vestibular issues. The child with gravitational insecurity should test out the chair when he is not scheduled for a procedure. A smaller child can simply sit in a parent's lap.

- Some children respond well to being wrapped gently while in the dentist chair. This should be voluntary. Tying a child onto a papoose board is unacceptable and traumatizing to the child who is already feeling out of control. If absolutely necessary, use mild sedation.

Doctor

With the fluorescent lighting, noisy paper on the examining table, tongue depressor, bright light in the eyes, and instruments looking in your nostrils and ears, plus vaccinations and blood draws, going to the doctor can be petrifying for any child. Follow the preparation advice for dentists given above—such as finding a friendly, patient doctor, visiting beforehand, observing another person being examined (but probably not receiving any needle sticks), reading books about going to the doctor, and role-playing doctor—so the child will know what to expect.

Here are a few additional tips:

- Ask whether there will be a long wait in the examining room. Do not have the child change into the gown until the doctor is actually ready to examine the child. If the office has crinkly paper gowns, have the child wear a soft, oversize man's shirt.

- Allow the child to listen to favorite music during the exam.

- Allow the child to wear a cap to shield against harsh lights.

- Give the child a security object item (a favorite toy, lucky charm) or weighted lap pad or weighted toy if that is soothing.

- While all kids hate getting shots and having blood drawn, most get over it fairly quickly. Other kids take hours, days, or even weeks to recover. To reduce some of the trauma, teach parents to:

  - Review a Social Story about blood draws. There's one good for any child at helpautismnow.com/blood_draw.html.

  - Ask the doctor about numbing the area prior to getting shots or having blood drawn via a prescription for lidocaine or EMLA cream (a lidocaine and prilocaine mixture) or an over-the-counter product such as Dr. Numb. These creams can be thickly layered on 45 minutes before to going to the doctor. Reapplication may be necessary if there is a long wait. The doctor may also be able to use a topical coolant spray or an ice pack to quickly lower skin temperature for a numbing effect.

  - Try Buzzy, a small vibrating bee with a unique ice pack which is designed to desensitize nerves (buzzy4shots.com).

  - Distract the child with a DVD on a portable player or an iPad during the procedure. Definitely reward the child for doing his or her best during the exam!

MRIs, Sleep Studies, and Other Procedures

MRI procedures are incredibly loud even for the person with typical hearing. Be sure to bring along earplugs to be worn in addition to the earmuffs the MRI technician will provide. Practice wearing the earplugs at home, as well as wearing snugly fitting headphones to approximate the MRI experience.

Help the child select a soothing, happy visualization to focus on during the procedure such as going to Disneyland, swimming with dolphins, or whatever the child loves thinking about. Speak with the doctor about a mild sedative if the child is unable to remain still during the procedure.

Some diagnostic procedures such as EEGs require placement of electrodes on the skin. Some kids are grossed out by the electrode conduction paste and the idea that the electrodes are going to be glued on for a period of time. As with other medical procedures, it's best to prepare the child for what is going to happen to eliminate the element of surprise. You can role-play electrode placement and review the Social Story available online at One Place for Special Needs (2013).

If the child is going to be staying overnight for a sleep study, it will take place in a private room, and a parent should spend the night there as well. Parents can bring familiar bedding, including pillow and sheets, pajamas, stuffed animals, or other comfort items. There is usually a television but parents may want to pack a portable video player just in case. YouTube has many videos about sleep studies that can be previewed with the child. As always, balance how much advance information will be reassuring versus how much will make the child anxious.

Taking Medicine and Supplements

Swallowing large pills and liquid medication like "pink stuff" (amoxicillin) can be very challenging for the child with sensory issues. Consider these strategies:

- Oral suspensions and some pills can be mashed up and mixed into formula, milk, fruit juice, ginger ale, or other cold drinks if taken immediately. Be sure to ask the doctor about this, especially if the pill is in time-release form.
- Many vitamins and nutritional supplements can be mixed into foods such as applesauce, oatmeal, peanut butter, and so on. Try it yourself first to make sure it tastes okay and recognize that a picky eater will notice something is different. It's usually best to be honest about what you've done. Again, check with your doctor.

- Ask the doctor about using a compounding pharmacy that can add flavorings to liquid medication or create lollipops and transdermal gels.

- To help a child, teen, or adult to swallow a pill, coat it in something yummy and slippery such as honey to help it slide down more easily. Teach the person to place it toward the very back of the tongue and have water or juice to wash it down immediately.

- Try an Oralflo Pill Swallowing Cup, which uses the natural swallowing reflex. Fill the cup halfway with juice or water, put the pill on the grille and drink naturally through the spout (available in most drugstores and at oralflo.com).

Sleep Time

Sensory issues can have a huge impact on sleep. And sleep, of course, can have a huge impact on everything.

An auditory-sensitive child may have trouble filtering out sounds, whether it's traffic outside, the TV down the hall, or even the sound of a sibling breathing in the next bed or next room. A tactile-defensive child may be bothered by the pajamas, sheets, pillow, blanket, or the firmness of the mattress. The room may be too warm, too cool, too bright, or too dark for the child to relax and sleep. Happily, fairly simple changes can make a big difference. The following are some suggestions for bedtime.

Establish a Routine

Have the child go to bed and wake up at the same time every morning, seven days a week. It's tempting to let kids stay up late and sleep late on weekends and vacations, but this confuses the body's internal time clock and can disrupt sleep well beyond the weekend or holiday. Should the sleep schedule get out of whack due to vacations, holidays, or travel, adjust it back toward the child's regular bedtime by approximately 15 minutes per day.

For kids who struggle with transitions and have a hard time going to bed, start the bedtime routine up to an hour in advance. Develop a sequence for getting ready for bed such as brushing teeth and washing face, talking about the day's events, reading a book, and then lights out. Build in some variety so the child doesn't get too rigid about bedtime rituals. A parent may always read a book, but it can be different books throughout the week. It may be comforting for kids to have a Social Story about the bedtime routine and, for some, to have a picture schedule for each step.

While we may assume that evening activities should be calm and quiet, some children actually require intense vestibular and proprioceptive input before they can settle in for the night. A parent may find that a child falls asleep more easily if, for example, he starts his routine by jumping on his mini-trampoline or climbing a few flights of stairs and then brushes his teeth, changes into pajamas, and so on.

A bath is often soothing for kids before bed because the water provides deep pressure. If the child does not drink bath water, a parent can try adding Epsom salts to the bath since the magnesium helps relax muscles and induce sleep. However, some kids are overstimulated by a bath just before bed. If this is the case, they should bathe earlier or in the morning.

Many kids and adults self-soothe orally. If the child craves chewing gum, sucks his thumb, bites himself, or puts nonfood objects in his mouth frequently, he may benefit from an oral comfort such as a Chewy Tube, Ark Grabber, KidCompanions Chewlery, or a Dr. Bloom's Chewable Jewel. You'll find these and more in therapy catalogs and online.

Make the Room, Clothing, and Bedding Comfy

Minimize environmental noise by keeping the house relatively quiet, using a white noise machine, CD, White Noise iPhone app, or fan, or actually soundproofing the room and installing double-pane windows. In noisy city apartments, extremely auditory-sensitive children—especially infants and recently adopted children—may need actual soundproof windows that entirely seal out noise from outside. These windows, available from companies such as citiquiet.com, are pricey but do not require alteration of existing windows which makes them good for renters and owners alike.

Use a nightlight or very dim table lamp if the child prefers one. At the same time, a sensitive child may sleep best in a room that is completely dark. The parent may need to install blackout shades and add weatherstripping around the bedroom door and a door flap on the bottom to prevent light from seeping in. A rolled-up towel works but makes it difficult for the child to get out during the night if needed.

Make sure the room isn't too hot or too cold. Do what you can do to fix vibrations from an air conditioner or a clanging radiator. Use a humidifier if the air is very dry or a dehumidifier if the air is humid. Consider an air purifier with a HEPA filter to reduce airborne allergens.

Most kids prefer all-cotton bedding and cotton or polar fleece pajamas with tags and labels removed and without elastic waistbands and cuffs. Kids, teens, and adults that get overheated during the night might like SHEEX moisture-wicking sheets, available from Bed Bath & Beyond.

Double-check that the mattress is not lumpy, too hard, or too soft. Some children get the tactile and body awareness input they need to fall asleep and stay asleep from a weighted blanket. Some kids love sleeping in a sleeping bag for some extra proprioceptive input. Many cute, inexpensive ones are available, such as the Sensory Sak (sensoryuniversity.com). You'll find lots of sleep time comfort items like sleeping bags, weighted blankets, vibrating pillows, the Cloud b Sleep Sheep and Twilight Turtle, and white noise machines and CDs online (and see sensoryprocessingchallenges.com).

Other Sleep Strategies

- Eliminate or reduce daytime naps because they may interfere with nighttime sleep.
- If the child is sensitive to smells, take out the garbage before bedtime and air out lingering cooking smells. Use unscented laundry detergent on bedding and pajamas and, in general, avoid fabric softener because it leaves a residue.
- Avoid having your child associate the bedroom with fun, wakeful activities. Reserve the bed for sleeping only.
- Redecorate with soothing colors and avoid patterned wallpaper, carpets, and linens if the child tends to get visually stimulated.

- Medications such as antihistamines, stimulants, and mood stabilizers can directly impact sleep. Work with the pediatrician or psychopharmacologist to establish the best dosing schedule for necessary medications. Avoid products with caffeine such as chocolate, hot cocoa, ice tea, colas, Mountain Dew, Midol, or Excedrin Migraine at least 6 hours before bed.

- Parents might consider a trial of synthetic melatonin. Melatonin is a hormone which is naturally secreted by the pineal gland which helps regulate sleep-wake cycles. Available in a spray or a pill, supplementation with melatonin has been found to be safe and often effective for children, including those with autism.

- Remind parents to use these sleep strategies themselves. A well-rested caregiver is far better than an exhausted one for helping a child get a good night's sleep.

Growing Up

Dealing with puberty presents a host of new challenges for kids with SPD and their families. Peer pressure, desire to fit in, and physical changes that come with growing up can be tricky. Advice from parents may be decidedly unwelcome, and peers may become more influential. Some kids simply don't care whether they fit in with the crowd and wear their differences like a badge of honor, but most kids want to fit in with their peers. The adolescent who never took off his sweatpants in grammar school may scramble to find blue jeans he can tolerate. The girl who avoided loud music may learn to at least pretend she likes the latest hit, though she might want to keep some earplugs handy or hidden behind her long hair.

The following are a few common obstacles and solutions for teens.

Body Odor

Due to differences in smell sensitivity, a sensory-impaired teen or young adult may be meticulous about always smelling nice and fresh or, conversely, may be oblivious to stinky socks and armpits. A person who would prefer that other people back off from him may use his personal phew factor to make this happen. Nevertheless, smelling okay is a basic social rule. Proliferation of bacteria is a hygiene issue and therefore nonnegotiable.

A person may find the feeling or odor of deodorant to be repellent. An individual may need to do some patient experimentation to find a deodorant that is acceptable, trying a variety of liquid roll-ons, dry cake roll-ons, and sprays. Unscented products are usually the best choice. Given the person's level of sensitivity, look for a deodorant that has minimal chemicals, particularly without aluminum chlorohydrate, a salt that is one of the most common ingredients in commercial antiperspirants. Many studies have examined the link between aluminum toxicity and Alzheimer's disease and breast cancer. While no definitive link has been found, it is safest to avoid applying aluminum to the body daily—or to wash it off at the end of the day at the very least.

There are many healthier products on the market such as Tom's of Maine, available at most health food stores, Whole Foods, and elsewhere, which may be more acceptable in terms of smell and texture. Exploration is key.

Shaving

Young men learning to shave will need to find the right combination of razor and shaving cream to shave sensitive facial skin. Girls wanting to shave their legs and armpits will also need to do some experimentation. Here are some ideas:

- Taking a hot shower first softens the hair, making it easier to shave.
- Cheap, disposable razors are more likely to irritate and nick the skin. Better to use a high-quality razor.
- Some may prefer electric razors that vibrate against the skin. Others find them more irritating.
- For some, the ritual of creating lather and applying it with a nice shaving brush and high-quality shaving soap is soothing.
- Using cake shaving soap and a brush eliminates the need to touch shaving cream directly.

Menstruation

An informed young woman is more confident when she gets her period. Whether to use a pad or tampon should depend on personal preference. A pad may be preferable during light flow days. To make tampon insertion more comfortable, she can use vaginal lubricant.

If the young woman has menstrual cramps, pain relief is important. Anti-inflammatory NSAIDs such as Advil and Aleve can be very helpful, especially if taken at the onset of cramps. If cramping is intense and if blood flow is very heavy, birth control pills may be considered. This discussion should take place between the teenager and a gynecologist or pediatrician who treats older girls. Parents should recognize that it's embarrassing and awkward for a teenager to be in the same waiting room as toddlers and infants. Heating pads can help too. At school, a young woman can wear a ThermaCare wrap that heats up mechanically and stays warm for up to 6–8 hours.

Girls have begun to menstruate much earlier within the past few decades, with obesity and environmental exposure to endocrine-disrupting chemicals such as pesticides, plastics, and hormones in food and cosmetic products suspected to play pivotal roles. A landmark study of over 17,000 girls found that black girls, on average, experience the first signs of puberty between ages 8 and 9 and that white girls experience these changes by age 10. This is two years earlier for black girls and one year earlier for white girls than had been found in prior studies. Precocious puberty is thus now defined as occurring before age 7 in black girls, age 8 in white girls, and before age 9 in boys (Herman-Giddens et al., 1997; Siddiqi, Van Dyke, Donohoue, & McBrien, 1999).

While nature must ultimately take its course, it may be advisable to delay the onset of puberty for girls who are between ages 3 and 6 and possibly between ages 6 and 8—or girls who are seriously not yet ready to handle the physical and psychosocial challenges of puberty and menstruation due to significant cognitive and behavioral challenges. Lupron is a hormone-suppressing drug injected monthly, which may be given until the normal age of puberty (ages 8–13 for girls and ages 9–14 for boys). Side effects of Lupron include bone density loss, hot flashes, and mood changes and should be monitored closely by a medical professional. Lupron therapy has been completely discredited for the specific treatment of autism.

Using Beauty Products

Parents may be surprised to find their daughter who cried when they put sun block on when she was little suddenly becomes interested in using beauty products because other girls do. Finding acceptable lotions and cosmetics takes some trial and error. Here are some tips:

- Health food stores are a good place to find unscented facial moisturizers, cosmetics that do not contain nasty chemicals, and toluene- and formaldehyde-free nail polish.

- Make beauty treatments at home using all-natural ingredients: organic food-grade coconut oil to deep-condition hair and soften cuticles; whipped egg white pore-tightening facial masks; soothing mashed cucumber masks to reduce puffiness; and honey facial masks to moisturize. These treatments are fun, inexpensive, and great for sensory exploration. You'll find plenty of recipes online.

- Girls should experiment with cosmetics if they are interested in wearing them. There is a big sensory difference, for example, between lip gloss and lipstick or powdered foundation and liquid foundation. Teach them KISS: Keep It Simple Sweetie and that less is more, but respect individual preferences.

- Remind girls that they should always remove any makeup before going to bed to keep skin clean and healthy. They should experiment with eye makeup remover cream versus liquids to find one that is acceptable.

- If teenaged girls and boys tend to get pimples, teach them to clean their faces carefully and to gently exfoliate facial skin at least once a week. Exfoliating treatments with smaller granules are usually best tolerated. Mud masks can help dry up oily pimple-prone skin. Chemical treatments such as Clearasil may be helpful, but irritating. Bioré strips may help to painlessly remove blackheads. If possible and well-tolerated, teens should get facials to help keep skin pores open.

Dating and Sex

Beginning to date is a rite of passage fraught with insecurity and delight for just about every teen. It is important that adolescents and young adults with sensory challenges learn to self-advocate for the kinds of intimate contact they do and do not enjoy. People who cannot endure light touch will need to learn to tell their partners about touch preferences, for example.

While many parents would like to have children abstain from dating and intimate relations until marriage (or forever!), this is simply not what happens for most teens and young adults. Therefore, like most social-emotional challenges, both dating and sex need to be discussed openly.

It may be worthwhile to articulate to teens that it is perfectly okay to wait to engage in intimate contact until they are sure they want to. Once sexual intimacy becomes a factor—even a potential factor—both males and females need information and access to reliable, tolerable means of birth control unless they are ready, in fact, to have a baby.

To avoid sexually transmitted diseases (STDs) such as AIDS, herpes, chlamydia, and gonorrhea, condoms must be used. Condoms may be quite unpleasant to use from a sensory standpoint. Gooey lubricant and weird-feeling material on sensitive skin can be a problem. It may take some trial and error to find the most tolerable brand. Latex condoms may be very irritating for some males and females alike, and should be avoided entirely by people with latex allergies. Recently developed polyisoprene condoms made of synthetic latex are a good alternative since they are softer and stretchier and often more comfortable than polyurethane condoms, another latex alternative. Polyisoprene condoms include LifeStyles Skyn or Durex Avanti. Lambskin condoms do not protect against STDs and should not be used.

CHAPTER 7

Working With Schools

School can be an oasis or an absolute nightmare for students with sensory processing issues. So much depends on goodness of fit between a student's sensory challenges, personality, and learning style and the school's educational approach, physical environment, and the chemistry with individual teachers and school staff members.

Most schools emphasize auditory and visual learning and reward students who learn best through these sensory modalities. A child who loves reading, listening to a teacher speaking at the front of the classroom, and working solo on projects will excel in a quiet, structured setting in which students sit at assigned desks and have clearly defined behavioral and academic expectations. The child who prefers physically active, hands-on learning will have difficulty sitting still and staying tuned in with his eyes and ears. He will likely fare better in a less structured classroom that includes more active student participation, working in groups, and lots of opportunities for physical exploration.

Even when the child is fortunate enough to be placed in a school setting that matches his or her needs well, going to school can magnify any sensory difficulties. All of those sensory quirks that parents may have learned to accommodate at home can become problems when a child goes to school. There is a huge difference between the familiar sights, sounds, smells, and other sensory input experienced at home and the unpredictable chaos inherent in an institutional environment with many unfamiliar adults and children and increased demands for good behavior and academic achievement.

At the first parent-teacher conference, a parent may be stunned to learn that a child who is easygoing and sweet at home is pushing other children, refusing to line up or help at clean-up time, and prefers looking at picture books alone in the corner to engaging in dress-up, using play dough, or block play with others.

Of course, some kids with sensory challenges do learn to buck up and summon up all of their psychic and physical energy to keep it together all day at school. These kids may be exhausted and simply fall apart when they get home each day.

The ability to handle sensory challenges at school varies from child to child, day to day, class to class, and sometimes moment to moment. Fortunately there are many sensory strategies that therapists, teachers, and students can use to make the school day more sensory friendly. As you read through this chapter, you'll get lots of ideas and strategies for helping children have a better experience at school. Many of them can be implemented informally with an understanding teacher or officially through either a 504 Plan or an IEP. Most often, sensory strategies are recommended by the school-based OT or private OT the family brings in on a consulting basis. The mental health clinician can play a key role, confirming the validity of sensory strategies for a particular child or personally implementing them if no OT is available.

INFORMAL ARRANGEMENTS

Quite often, sensory strategies can be implemented immediately with an understanding classroom teacher or paraprofessional. She may readily see how taking quick movement breaks throughout the day helps certain students stay on task much better or may be more than happy to give certain students preferential seating if that helps them to listen better. She may love the idea of passing out hand fidgets during circle time and dimming the lights or playing gentle music rather than raising her voice to quiet students or to warn them of an upcoming transition.

Staff development days are a great time to teach the teachers about sensory processing issues and how to accommodate a wide variety of sensory needs in the classroom. Recommendations for a particular student should be personalized, although no one child should be singled out for special treatment. If Sally will benefit from sitting on an inflatable wedge cushion in order to maintain upright posture while getting a little dynamic movement through her hips and trunk, it is simple enough to provide a wedge cushion. Ideally, several wedge cushions will be available in the classroom.

In an informal arrangement, the school is not obligated to purchase any equipment on behalf of a student or to implement a sensory strategy. In order for the piece of equipment—be it a seat cushion, chair, molded pencil grip, slant board—or any modification of the school environment or activities to be mandatory, it needs to be recorded in a legal document—a 504 Plan or IEP.

504 PLANS

A 504 Plan is a legal document that specifies the school's obligations to accommodate a student with special needs. A 504 Plan is actually based on Section 504 of the Rehabilitation Act of 1973, which protects the rights of students who have physical or mental impairments, do not qualify for special education, and yet still need assistance.

A 504 Plan may include accommodations such as medication administration; test and assignment modifications such as extended time, or answers recorded in any manner (e.g., using a computer or dictating material to a scribe); adaptive seating such as an inflatable cushion or special chair; adjustments to environment such as being allowed to eat lunch in a room other than the cafeteria; and so on. Generally, a parent must make an official request for a 504, and OTs, school psychologists, neuropsychologists, or other clinicians may recommend that the parent do so.

A child who receives any special education services should have an Individualized Education Program (IEP), not a 504 Plan.

IEPS

The IEP is a legal document required by the Individuals With Disabilities Education Act (IDEA), a federal law enacted in 1975 that requires public schools to provide special education services for children with disabilities. IDEA is based on the premise that children with disabilities are entitled to a free and appropriate public education in the least restrictive environment. This means children should be taught in regular education classrooms rather than in special education classrooms whenever possible and provided with the accommodations they need in order to do so.

Under IDEA, the school district is required to provide an appropriate education, not necessarily the very best one possible for any individual child. Parents and schools may have very different definitions of "appropriate" and sometimes there is a clash between what is offered by the school in terms of educational setting and therapeutic and support services and what the parent believes the child actually needs. This is can be especially true for the student with sensory processing difficulties which some school administrators have never even heard of.

It may be necessary for a parent to explain what sensory issues are and how they impact the child's performance at school. Keep in mind that difficulties at home such as resistance to taking a shower, getting a haircut, getting dressed, and going to parties are not going to earn your child services and accommodations at school. Difficulties tolerating noisy environments such as the cafeteria due to auditory hypersensitivity, vestibular underreactivity requiring frequent, brief movement breaks, and adaptive seating during circle time due to low muscle tone and body awareness deficits are just a few concrete examples of how a child's sensory issues can directly impact school performance. Once the impact of sensory issues on the child's ability to access the educational curriculum is clearly articulated, then you, the family, and the school are ready to make a plan for how to meet those needs.

The IEP is the document that will serve as a road map for making this happen. For the child who receives special ed services, the IEP must spell out specifics such as school accommodations (preferential seating, sensory diet activities, and others), assistive technology, therapeutic and educational goals, and mandates for related services such as occupational, physical, and speech therapy.

Many parents are under the impression that if their child receives OT services at school, it will address their child's sensory processing difficulties. Of course, school-based OT is not the same as going to an OT clinic or dedicated sensory gym. It is important to remember that school-based services such as OT, PT, and speech therapy are simply intended to support the student's ability to meet IEP goals.

IEP goals should be developed collaboratively by a multidisciplinary team of educators and therapists to identify the activities and behaviors the student needs to achieve in order to succeed in the educational program. Sensory diet and self-regulation techniques are intervention strategies that can be incorporated to accomplish educational goals.

Seek out the expertise and active participation of every related service provider who works with the student. For example, if the child misbehaves during transitions between classes, the PT should have input regarding goals related to ambulation and stair climbing, the OT may recommend accommodations regarding visual processing skills due to lighting and depth perception challenges, and the speech therapist may help the student to communicate his discomfort and to advocate for himself.

Make sure the child's IEP goals and objectives are SMART: Specific, Measurable, Action words, Realistic, and Time-specific so it is possible to track progress. There is a big difference between saying, "Noah will improve his self-regulation skills" and "Following heavy work and breathing exercises, Noah will focus on tabletop tasks for 10 minutes with one verbal prompt."

IEP Meeting Tips That Empower Parents

The key to a successful IEP meeting is to go in prepared. Therapists can review these tips with parents to help ensure the meeting proceeds successfully.

- Read your child's current IEP and consider what is and is not working. Make a list of issues you want to address and questions you want to ask. Take careful notes or bring along someone who can take notes for you while you listen. Consult with a parent advocate or lawyer who specializes in special education issues if need be.

- Request a copy of all school assessments prior to the meeting and bring along copies of any evaluation reports done outside of school. Ask the school for proposed recommendations prior to the meeting so you know what to expect.

- The IEP meeting notice sent from the school must include a list of attendees. Parents are entitled to invite school-based service providers as well as outsiders such as private mental health clinicians and OTs or PTs. They should let the school know if they plan to bring anyone from outside the school such as a parent advocate, private therapist, or outside evaluator so they can be added to the list. If the people the parents want to attend the meeting are not available at the scheduled time, the meeting can be rescheduled.

- A special education and general education teacher must be in the room if the child spends any part of the day in one of those settings. Remember that everyone who signs in for the meeting has to stay for the duration. They cannot sign the document and leave.

- Make sure the meeting is about your child who has been diagnosed with a disability and creating an educational program that fits his or her unique needs. It is not about whether or not the law is fair or whether any special accommodations are convenient or too costly for the school district.

- If the child may need to use assistive technology, the IEP meeting is the time to request an assessment. Make sure this is marked off on the assistive technology box.

- Keep accommodations and strategies generic. For example, the IEP might specify that your child has the right to use an assistive technology device to take class notes rather than naming a specific item such as a Livescribe SmartPen. This way if his needs or the technology used changes you won't need to amend the IEP.

- While everyone is too busy these days, do not allow yourself to be rushed through the IEP process. A second meeting can be scheduled if necessary to make sure everything is sufficiently discussed and handled.

- Don't sign anything until you are completely satisfied with the arrangements. Make sure that everything mutually agreed to during the meeting is on the final IEP document. Don't let anyone bully you.

- Keep calm, polite, and cooperative, even if you are furious (which hopefully you won't be). Anger backfires every time. Review breathing and self-calming techniques before the meeting.

SENSORY SCENARIOS

Gabriella Goes to School

Gabriella hates to get up in the morning to go to school. Mom tries waking her up gently and slowly but usually winds up losing patience after a lot of cajoling. Gabriella doesn't like getting her face wet, but Mom makes her wash up and brush her teeth with that nasty minty paste. Just the smell of breakfast makes her nauseous, but she will nibble on a corn muffin. She gets on the school bus and covers her ears. Why do children always yell and scream in the morning? she asks herself. Why is the bus ride so bumpy and why does it stink like gasoline? Finally, she arrives at school along with hundreds of other students. It's morning mayhem in the school lobby. She finally gets to her classroom. Ugh, free choice time. Kids are pulling out blocks, Legos, and other toys from shelves. Gabriella selects a picture book and sits in her cubby. She looks up and sees the teacher setting up the day's special activity that includes painting. She sighs. It's going to be another long day at preschool.

Jesse's Lunchtime

Jesse is having an excellent day at school. He aced his math and spelling tests. He's really hungry by noon but waits for his classmates to get their food first. It's hard to balance that cafeteria tray loaded down with food. At least he learned to put a book on the seat closest to the food line so he doesn't have to walk far with his tray while searching for a seat. He gobbles down his food as quickly as he can so he's ready to line up for recess. As his second grade class is going outside, a classmate calls him Messy Jesse once again. He runs to the bathroom and sees he has crumbs all over his face. He notices that his shirt is on inside out again today. Jeez, who really cares anyway? he thinks and then wonders whether the other boys will let him join in the basketball game today.

Pete's Phys Ed Class

Thank goodness, Pete thinks. At last I can get out of this hard chair and move in physical education class. Who knew high school was going to have so much sitting and writing? The phys ed teacher this year is a problem though. He's tough. The minute Pete goes into the gym, he has to sit down and be quiet once again. Seriously! Then the teacher blah blah blahs and that wood floor is way too hard to sit on. And there are those cool ropes to climb. He's just aching to stand up and stretch. Oh my—new soccer balls. The phys ed teacher tells him to sit back down. Uh, okay. As the teacher blahs on, Pete stands up again. His backside hurts and then that's it: he's being sent to the principal's office again. Not fair!

SCHOOL SOLUTIONS

If the child or teen is receiving occupational therapy services in school, he should be observed by the OT and helped to thrive in every school setting. If a child is working with an OT outside of school, he should also be assisted in a variety of school scenarios. The rest of this chapter will help the clinician understand many common school-based sensory processing issues and what can be done to help.

Starting the School Day

Many schools have staggered dropoff and pickup times to minimize the mayhem when children first arrive at school as well as when they go home. This can make a huge difference for the student who is overwhelmed by the noisy and busy movements of large groups of people.

If possible, the school can arrange for a sensitive child to arrive a few minutes early so he can easily go to his classroom to settle in right away. Alternately, the student may be allowed to go to a special place such as the main office or a therapist's room until most students are situated in their classrooms.

Other options to be discussed with parents include providing the student with sensory diet input prior to school as well as ear protection and an action plan.

- Sensory diet activities prior to school may include a firm massage or squishy hugs while still in bed; playing favorite music as part of a wake-up routine; jumping on a mini trampoline, spinning on a dizzy disk, wheelbarrow walking to the bathroom, taking the stairs instead of the elevator, or another movement activity that helps wake up the body and brain to help set the tone for a good day at school.

- Carbohydrates for breakfast, especially sugared carbs, provide little nutritional value. Even TV commercials clearly state that breakfast cereals are just part of a nutritious breakfast. A bowl of Cap'n Crunch with some milk gives a child instant energy, but does not provide enough nutritive value to carry the child through the morning. Some kind of protein to feed the nervous system before school will serve the child well. It does not have to be traditional breakfast fare. If the child loves chicken nuggets with cheese, that's fine. A fruit smoothie, perhaps with some whey powder added, is a wonderful healthy breakfast drink.

While riding the school bus, taking a subway, or entering the crowded school lobby at dropoff time, the child can wear sound-reducing earmuffs such as those by Peltor or other brands; Sensgard's lightweight hearing protectors that look like headphones with plugs which block sound from entering the ear by covering the outside of the ear canal; or traditional sound-reducing earplugs from a drugstore or online (at places like earplugstore.com). The child might listen to preferred music over headphones at home or on the way to and/ or from school. The child may be able to self-regulate by holding a favored hand fidget tool such as a squeeze ball or worry stone. Likewise, wearing a weighted vest or compression may be comforting and organizing at these times.

Unstructured Play Time

Lots of children love the open-ended freedom of choice time, gravitating toward favorite toys and activities, whether it's building an elaborate structure out of blocks, doing imaginative play with buddies, pouring and mixing at the sand table, or drawing with markers and crayons. Many young students with sensory issues become overwhelmed by all the sights, sounds, and movement in the classroom and struggle with purposeful exploration of classroom toys and equipment.

Children who are oversensitive to stimuli tend to wind up engaged in solitary play on the sidelines. They may seek out the same doll or toy truck each time, engaging in repetitive and self-absorbed play in a quiet area of the room. They may mosey around from one exploration station to the next looking at what others are doing for a minute or two, or simply wander aimlessly around the periphery of the room. They may refuse to help at cleanup time because they cannot tolerate being in the midst of what they perceive as chaos and confusion.

Children who are undersensitive or sensory cravers tend to seek out movement and deep pressure input, grabbing up blocks and hurling them, crashing into other kids, pounding on toys. They may need frequent reminders to be gentle, to keep their hands to themselves, and to watch where they are going. They may play with one toy for just one or two minutes before jumping over to the next one. During cleanup time, they may have trouble following directions and become overexcited and overstimulated.

It helps to impose some structure on the student who doesn't know what to do with herself during these open-ended periods. A parent or teacher may help the child who is "lost in space" during choice time to select what she is going to do beforehand. The child may benefit from a written list of activities, perhaps with a drawing or photo of the toys or equipment she will use. Then she can cross off each item once she has completed it. The point is to get the child engaged in class-room activities and routines, not necessarily to complete the full list. If the child is having a blast doing some beading or driving toy trucks, the mission is accomplished. The list is there for backup for when the child becomes defocused.

For the sensory-seeking child, such a list should consist of several organizing, self-regulating activities that satisfy the child's craving for sensory input so he can participate in group play in an adaptive way. This may include doing intense movement and body awareness activi-ties such as jumping on a trampoline or doing jumping jacks, som-ersaults, wall and floor push ups, animal-themed yoga stretches, or using a Body Sock—a Lycra/Spandex sack the child can climb inside and stretch into a variety of shapes for strong deep pressure and body awareness.

Using Timers

Remember that kids have a notoriously poor sense of time. For kids who are engaged and having fun, free play may seem to go by in a matter of minutes. For the child who struggles with open-ended play, it may seem to drag on forever. A timer lets the child know how much time she has to play—or tolerate being in a boring situation. It may help the younger student to have a visual timer to help him gauge time as it passes, such as the Time Timer, which works really well for children who cannot yet read a clock or who need a quick visual to see how much time is left.

Getting a sense of time and understanding how every minute counts can help students immensely. The busy child who has trouble initiating an academic task may procrastinate by sharpening his pen-cil, going to the bathroom, getting a tissue, getting a drink of water, and only then sitting down and getting to work—and then complain that he didn't have enough time to complete his work. An appropriate timer will provide a visual of time that disappears as it elapses, which can be quite helpful for taking tests, writing in-class essays, giving oral presentations, choice time, and more.

The Time Timer, an excellent choice for schools, comes in several versions: a wristwatch for older students; a 3-inch timer for personal use; a 12-inch timer most people can see from across the room; iPad, iPhone, and Android apps; and desktop computer software. Set for up to one hour (or customized for longer periods on the apps and software), the Time Timer's signature red disk disappears as time elapses, helping everyone see how much time is left. Most models have an optional auditory alarm as well.

Another great visual timer is the Learning Resources Time Tracker, which functions like a traffic light to tell kids at a glance whether they have plenty of time (green light), need to starting to wind down (yellow light), and when it's time to stop (red light). There are accompanying tones for each color. Old-fashioned egg timers can also work well.

If children are not too startled by sudden sounds, alarms on the iPhone and other mobile devices can be set to fun sounds such as a guitar strum, quacking duck, or motorcycle.

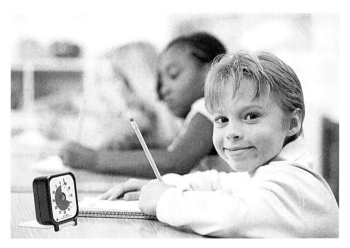

The Time Timer helps kids visualize time as it passes. *Photo courtesy of Time Timer LLC*

Circle Time

Many young students struggle to sit still and remain attentive at circle time or meeting time on the floor for reasons including these:

- Low muscle tone and floppy muscles cannot fight the force of gravity well enough to hold the child upright for any length of time.
- Decreased muscular strength, especially in abdominals and back extensor muscles, results in muscle fatigue when held in static, unchanging contractions.
- Poor body awareness due to poor proprioceptive processing results in difficulty managing body position in space.
- Difficulty processing auditory and visual input makes looking at and listening to the teacher and filtering out other sounds increasingly tiresome as time passes.
- Tactile issues make sitting on a hard floor or thin carpeting painful while sitting so close to classmates poses a risk of unwanted light touch.

Many adults have these issues too, especially poor core postural strength. No wonder so many teachers sit in chairs during circle time!

"Crisscross applesauce" (cross-legged sitting) is especially difficult for a child with low muscle tone, loose ligaments, poor body awareness, and other issues. These kids will melt into the floor with the top of the pelvis tilting back (posterior pelvic tilt), the spine forming a C-curve, and the neck hyperextended so that the child can look up and see what's going on. If you try it yourself, you will see how unpleasant it is. Slump way down wherever you are sitting so that you are hunched over. Now look up and notice what it's like to see, swallow, and breathe. This dysfunctional position can result in backaches and neck aches, and interfere with respiration and digestion.

Most students with these issues will compensate somehow—either by sitting in a more stable though unacceptable position or by changing body position frequently. Many young children with poor muscle tone and strength along with loose ligaments in the joints of their lower extremities learn early on which body position offers the most stable base of support. W-sitting with internally rotated hips and weight on knees and ankles provides a very wide sitting base and lots of proprioceptive input to the body since the child bears weight not only on the pelvic bones, but also through the entire lower extremities: hips, femurs, knees, lower leg, ankles, and feet. While W-sitting is quite stable for the child, it is not good for development since it causes stress to the hip and knee joints, inhibits trunk rotation and core muscles, and interferes with crossing the body's midline. Other children will switch from crisscross to long-legged sitting to ring sitting to kneeling to flopping around on their backs or tummies so that different postural muscles are engaged and no one set of muscles gets fatigued. Moving around also helps the child get more proprioceptive and vestibular input in an attempt to stay alert.

Schools should carefully consider at what age and for how long children should be expected to sit on the floor. Toddlers should not be required to sit in circle time until they are 36 months old (Copple & Bredekamp, 2009). As many children with special needs have significant lags in development, the age when sitting on the floor for circle time is developmentally appropriate or even possible may be much later. Preschool circle time should run 10–15 minutes, depending on the ability of the particular group of students to sit and attend. Amazingly, some preschool circle times run for 30 minutes or longer, usually inappropriate cognitively and physically. Meeting time for older students may also last longer than many students can comfortably tolerate.

The following are some strategies and accommodations teachers can make to help students during circle time and meeting time.

Duration and Timing

Schedule circle time or meeting time soon after gross motor activity periods such as recess or gym class. If this is not possible, teachers can incorporate fun physical activities beforehand to provide intense vestibular and proprioceptive input. If this is not possible, circle time should at the very least begin with at least two minutes of movement such as "shaking the sillies out." Some teachers may be concerned that this will rev up students exactly when they need to be calm and quiet. In practice, it works quite the opposite, because jazzing up the muscles by stretching, bouncing, jumping, hopping, running, and other types of movement input helps to reset bodies and brains, enabling students to sit and tune in with their ears and eyes. You'll find movement activities that can easily be incorporated into the classroom later in this chapter.

Spatial Considerations

Most students benefit from external cues that organize them in space, and kids with sensory issues often need extra help in this area. Teachers can provide students with visual place markers that help them know where their bodies belong. Laminated paper mats with the child's name or photo attached to a defined circle will help children learn how to form a circle and know exactly where they belong at any given time. Carpet squares may work even better to create body boundaries, plus kids get nice sensory input from picking up and carrying carpet squares from a different part of the room to the circle area. Most will appreciate the added cushioning under their bottoms on the hard floor. Those who need to can fidget with the carpeting as long as hands remain on their own square. Teachers can add ribbons or fabric tabs to the edges if needed. Finally the space should be large enough so that children do not have to squeeze together to fit and deal with unwanted bumps and nudges.

Children who have difficulty with visual or auditory attention should be positioned carefully in the teaching space, usually close to the teacher. At the same time, a child who dislikes casual, unexpected touch may need to be situated so that she knows there is nobody behind her. Often positioning her by the wall or a bookcase will give a little extra space away from classmates and some added security.

Seating Considerations

Some students will continue to need help meeting their body's natural need for frequent movement (Ishihara, Dake, Kashihara, & Ishihara, 2010). These students may benefit from a lightly inflated seat cushion that is designed to improve sitting posture. One such cushion that is very popular in some schools is the Disc 'O' Sit, which allows students to remain seated while they subtly wiggle (Pfeiffer, Henry, Miller, & Witherell, 2008). For kids who slump, a wedge-shaped cushion called the Movin' Sit can help correct the position of the pelvis and spine when the wide end is placed toward the back (see photo, page 174). It is essential to not overinflate these cushions because that will destabilize the student just when he needs added stability. A vibrating sitting pillow may provide input that helps a child sit still comfortably (senseez.com).

Children who have more significant difficulty with floor sitting— those who W-sit for stability, have a spinal C-curve, or move continuously—may need greater physical support. Students may sit much more comfortably on dense foam yoga blocks, plastic cube chairs, low benches, or specially designed floor sitters that provide back support. Sitting kids against the wall or a bookcase will help a little bit, but it does not provide adequate support for the child with neuromuscular or proprioceptive issues. The BackJack chair is a popular classroom choice, with a Movin' Fit wedge cushion added for students who need help with their sitting posture.

Kids that seek out tactile and proprioceptive input by leaning against others, lying down, or rolling around on the floor may benefit from sitting in a bean bag chair or wearing a CuddleLoop or homemade Lycra wrap, which snugly swaddles the student when he sits and gives sensory feedback as he makes postural adjustments. A HowdaHug chair is a nice option too. This floor sitter, composed of wooden slats, provides compression and may be cushioned by adding an optional faux sheepskin zip-on cover. A variety of floor sitters are worth exploring online, in therapy and school supply catalogs, and even in some sporting goods stores.

Some students will participate much better if they do not sit on the floor at all. With its convex base and soft foam padding, the Hokki Stool (kaplanco.com) lets students move in all directions while remaining seated, which can help the child who needs to be physically active to stay tuned in. Other kinds of seating such as regular classroom chairs, ball chairs, rocking chairs, and other special chairs should also be considered at circle time if they enable students to access what is being taught.

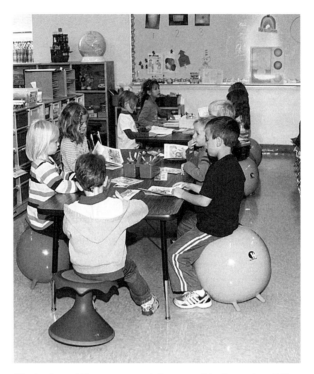

Students get the movement they need to focus by sitting on either stability balls or the Hokki stool. *Photo Courtesy of WittFitt LLC*

Circle time or meeting time may be the perfect time for a student to wear a weighted vest, lap pad, shoulder wrap, or other item (see Chapter 4) if it helps that child feel more organized and comfortable. As noted earlier, while there are recommendations for use of weighted wearables (but not for compression garments), the student should be allowed to wear the weighted vest or lap pad for the duration of the activity she is engaged in. Never interrupt a focused, productive child to put on or take off a weighted or compression garment.

Satisfy Busy Hands and Mouths

Hand fidgets and oral comforts often help kids stay tuned in during sitting time, whether on the floor or a chair, regardless of age. Teachers may provide a basket or bucket of hand fidget tools for the entire class, preferably topically related. Almost any classroom item will do—Cuisenaire rods, Unifix cubes, Koosh or squeeze balls, Silly Putty, and so on. Students may be allowed to bring their own fidget tools from home. Note that these are tools, not toys, and should be treated as such. No throwing or being silly with them. If a student is unable to resist throwing the fidget or drops it frequently, whether accidentally or on purpose, it can be attached to a belt loop with a lanyard and clip.

We all comfort ourselves orally, starting at birth. Oral comforts can include sipping water from an open cup or, for more sensory input, from a bottle with a sports nozzle. Students can bring in their own BPA-free plastic or stainless steel water bottles. Crunchy and chewy snacks such as carrot sticks, pretzels, dehydrated string beans, fruit leather, and chewing gum give lots of satisfying and organizing oral sensory input.

Chewing Gum

Studies show that chewing gum increases alertness and reduces chronic (but not acute) stress and enhances cognition (Allen & Smith, 2011). When we chomp on a piece of gum, we get lots of proprioceptive input into the joints of the jaw and teeth (gomphoses— the joints between each tooth and its bony socket). This movement also stimulates the oral motor muscles as well as the muscles and connective tissue on the scalp and neck. This sensory stimulation can be very helpful in helping students to focus.

While flavor preference is highly idiosyncratic, most kids like fruit-flavored gum. Kids who are understimulated as well as sensory seekers often enjoy strongly flavored gums such as spicy cinnamon. Ideally, avoid gums with artificial sweeteners such as aspartame. Glee Gum has no artificial colors or flavors and is gluten-free, casein-free for kids with celiac disease or who are simply sensitive to these proteins found in dairy, wheat, and other foods. Spry Gum and PÜR Gum are both very chewy and do not contain artificial sweeteners or artificial coloring. Both contain xylitol, a sugar alcohol sweetener that has been found to aid digestion and help prevent tooth decay.

Some schools outlaw chewing gum because students use it irresponsibly—spitting it on the floor or placing unwrapped chewed gum

under tabletops or in unlined garbage cans. Sometimes it's the custo-
dial crew that has insisted on a no-gum policy. This is a real shame,
and the policy is definitely worth revisiting as schools and classrooms
that allow gum chewing often have great results.

Desk Time

Sitting at a table or desk for sustained periods can be difficult for
the child, teen, or adult with sensory challenges. Issues with muscle
tone and strength and poor body awareness coupled with problems
staying still, ocular motor skills and visual acuity, hypersensitivity to
overhead lights, auditory discrimination deficits, tactile sensitivity
to materials used, and other factors can make sitting still and focusing draining or even next to impossible for some. Because of sensory problems, a child may wind up having problems with attention
and, therefore, learning. For others though, sitting at a table, working
independently, and listening quietly may be a welcome respite during
the school day.

Seating Considerations

To improve the seating experience for the student with sensory
issues, consider these strategies:

- Before having students sit down, engage the class in motor work
  and vestibular activities (see Easy Movement Ideas for the Classroom later in this chapter).

- Make sure the chair and table are appropriate to the student's
  size. When seated, the student's forearms and hands should rest
  comfortably on the tabletop so he does not have to hike up his
  shoulders in order to work on the surface. Hips, knees, and ankles
  should be at more or less right angles with feet able to be flat on
  the floor.

- Chair depth should match the distance from the student's back
  to a few inches behind the knees when seated. The front edge of
  the seat should never dig into the soft area behind the knee. At
  the same time, the child should be able to gain postural support
  from the back of the chair. If the seat is too deep (too much space

between the child's back and the back of the chair), a chair that provides lumbar (lower back) support should be found. At the very least, a cushion should be provided behind the child's back.

- If the child's feet cannot reach the floor, add a footrest. This can be an inexpensive footstool with a rubberized base (from Ikea and elsewhere), Just Foam blocks (from therapy catalogs), or even a yoga block with nonskid matting taped on. The Movin' Step inflatable footrest is a good option for a student who pushes against the front legs of his desk, because he can instead push down into this cushion. It is available in many therapy and exercise catalogs. Another solution for students who kick or push against desk legs is to tie a strip of Theraband or Lycra across the front chair legs for the student to push against.

- Just as when sitting on the floor, the student's pelvis, hips, and other body parts must be in a proper position to promote erect posture. There are several options to help, including these:

  - A lightly inflated seat cushion (e.g., Disc 'O' Sit or Swiss Disc) which provides a dynamic sitting surface that lets sitters subtly move to keep postural muscles activated while remaining stationary.

  - A Movin' Sit wedge-shaped cushion, which, when lightly inflated, helps to shift a posteriorly tilted pelvis into a more neutral position while providing an active seating surface.

  - Memory foam, meditation cushions, and molded seat cushions, which can also promote good posture and make sitting on a hard chair more comfortable.

- Some students actually do well with less support that forces them to activate postural muscles. A ball chair is a popular option for kids who are able to remain regulated and focused if they are able to move (Illi, 1994). A ball chair has a cuplike base that cradles a large therapy ball. Some styles have armrests. An appropriately sized ball may be also be used directly on the floor (some styles come with feet) for sitting. The Hokki Stool mentioned earlier is a good choice for this. Another option is a T-stool, composed of a seat on one vertical support that can be fabricated or purchased in therapy catalogs.

- A child who needs more sensory input to stay calm and focused may benefit from having a hand fidget tool at his desk, as discussed previously. If the child sits at a desk she will use for the entire school year, textured materials can be attached on the undersurface of the desk such as a strip of stick-on Velcro (both softer and rougher sides). Hand fidgets can be attached to desk legs so that they are always available and can be used without distracting classmates. Chewing gum, highly recommended if allowed, can help the seated student stay tuned in as well.

• Some students do best standing up, which lets them obtain vestibular input and burn off extra energy and calories. In light of this, some schools now offer students standing desks such as the AlphaBetter Stand-Up Desk (worthingtondirect.com) that lets kids stand or sit and swing their legs silently on a foot bar.

Use your best judgment about singling out any one student. Sensory tools such as inflatable seat cushions, hand fidgets, and water bottles can benefit all students and should be available for others to use as well.

Preferential Seat Location

Where the sensitive student sits can strongly influence how he attends and learns. It may be hard for a sensitive student to search for a seat when he enters a classroom since dealing with kids talking, walking, and jostling each other may make it difficult to visually scan for an available chair or make a good seat choice. The student with sensory issues may greatly appreciate having an assigned seat even if he travels to different rooms throughout the day.

The preferred seat location is often at the front of the classroom where the student's view is unobstructed and he has fewer distractions. Often it is reassuring to sit by a wall and away from the glare of light streaming in through windows. It should also be away from clanging radiators and whirring air conditioners. It may take some trial and error to find the best seat for an individual student in each classroom.

For the older student who travels from room to room, individual teachers can save a preferred seat to make the transition into each classroom easier. The science teacher, for example, can stack workbooks or graded papers on the student's table and thus reserve it for him without advertising it to the entire class.

Easy Movement Ideas for the Classroom

Frequent movement breaks boost learning and mood by stimulating sensory receptors, increasing oxygen intake, and releasing excess energy in a beneficial way. Having an opportunity to move is especially important in helping students get ready for classwork requiring sustained attention and at times of transition from one activity to another. Breaks may consist of activities such as jumping jacks, wall push-ups, chair push-ups, downward-facing dog and other yoga postures, stretching ("reach for the sky, reach for the earth"), marching around the room, and more. Here are a few additional ideas:

- Heavy work using large, deep muscles: do pushing, pulling, and carrying tasks such as moving furniture, pulling a wagon full of books, carrying a heavy bag, playing tug-of-war, catching a weighted ball, climbing stairs, wheelbarrow walking, and commando crawling.

- Play structured movement games such as selecting cards from Move Your Body, Upper Body and Core Strength, and/or Yogarilla Fun Decks (superduperinc.com).

- Assign special errands to students who need extra movement, such as carrying a note to the main office or distributing worksheets or supplies.

- Brain Gym activities get wiggles out, reduce stress, and help stimulate brain function. Some recommended Brain Gym activities include:

  - Brain buttons: This activity relaxes the neck and shoulders, helps balance right and left sides of the body, and boosts energy and focus. "Brain buttons" are the soft connective tissue pockets beneath your right and left collarbones. Place one hand on your belly while you massage these points with the thumb and middle finger of an outstretched hand for 20 to 30 seconds. Reverse hand placement and repeat.

  - Cross crawl: This activity increases communication between the left and right brain hemispheres and coordinates body sides. Start with "unilateral" (same side) movements (e.g., alternate right hand to right knee then left hand to left knee) and then do "contralateral" (opposite side) movements (e.g., alternate right hand to left knee, left hand to right knee, hand to foot in front of body, hand to foot behind body, and other variations).

- Lazy 8s: This activity loosens up arm muscles while focusing the brain. This is especially helpful when preparing to write. Hold your arm out with a pointed index finger and draw the infinity sign, a sideways 8. Draw it in the air using large arm movements, and keep the midpoint at the midline of your body so that your arm has to cross your midline. Next, draw it on paper. First use your dominant hand, drawing it quickly and loosely. Then, use your nondominant hand. To learn more Brain Gym activities you can easily incorporate into your practice, read *Brain Gym: Teacher's Edition* or take a course listed at braingym.org.

• MeMoves is a multimedia program that incorporates music, movement, and images, based on simple, geometric shapes students create with their bodies. It appeals to a wide range of ages and abilities and is very relaxing and engaging for students (see thinkingmoves.com).

• Use a high-quality mini-trampoline or rebounder with a stabilizing safety bar for younger students (needak.com) or a Bounce Pad or Bounce Disc (southpawenterprises.com).

• Teach students to breathe.

- Have students use straws, blow toys, and whistles.

- Teach deep, slow breathing, focusing on exhaling rather than inhaling. Younger students can roar like lions to exaggerate the exhale and thus breathe more deeply.

- Set up bowls of soapy water and straws and have students exhale forcefully through the straws to make "bubble mountains." They can hum as they exhale for even more fun deep breathing.

Lighting Considerations

Some people who are sensitive to light and sound are able to see and hear the flickering of fluorescent lights as the voltage switches on and off. This is more common for older fixtures that cycle on and off 60 times per second, while newer lights cycle significantly faster. However, even the newer fluorescents can be distracting and even disabling for the sensitive student. Fluorescent lighting has been associated with drowsiness, poor concentration, stress, eyestrain, headaches, and migraines (Basso, 2001; Martel, 2003).

Here's another thing to consider when using fluorescent lights. Compact fluorescents and other fluorescent lightbulbs contain a small amount of mercury sealed within the glass tubing. When a fluorescent bulb breaks, some mercury is released as mercury vapor. To minimize exposure to mercury vapor, the EPA provides recommended cleanup and disposal steps for hazardous materials (epa.gov/cfl/cflcleanup.html).

The simple fact is that any downcast lighting can be problematic for sensitive individuals. Add a ceiling fan and you'll get a strobe effect that may be highly uncomfortable for some people and may pose a risk to those prone to photoreactive seizures.

To improve lighting for all students and teachers, overhead fluorescent lights should be replaced with fixtures that contain, preferably, full-spectrum bulbs that cast off even, pleasant, illumination. If fluorescent fixtures absolutely cannot be replaced, turn them off and use floor lamps that can be bolted to walls for safety if necessary. For any kind of tabletop work or reading, a floor lamp that casts light from behind is best. Certainly in therapy rooms and resource rooms, students should work under lighting that is the most conducive to learning and a sense of well-being.

If it is not possible to make any modifications to fluorescent fixtures, be sure the lights have fresh fluorescent tubes that flicker less. Diffusers can be added to soften up the light. There are several light diffusers that comply with fire prevention guidelines, including inexpensive Classroom Light Filters (educationalinsights.com), festive, colorful Cozy Shades (schoolspecialty.com), and pricey but attractive U.S. Sky Panels (usaskypanels.com), which come in designs such as cherry blossoms and blue sky with fluffy clouds.

Curtains, shades, or sheers should be hung over windows to filter out glare, which can range from annoying to blinding. Installing dimmer switches is also ideal so brightness can be adjusted as needed to accommodate incoming light from outdoors.

Photosensitive students should be entitled to wear tinted lenses indoors if that enables them to see more comfortably. Optical-quality sunglasses and hats or visors with wide brims should be encouraged for outdoors, using Croakies or a neoprene strap if needed to hold them in place.

Noise Considerations

Due to large class sizes and avoidance of sound-absorbing fabrics such as carpeting due to sanitary concerns, many classrooms are way too loud for everyone. Teachers may find that they need to raise their voices to get attention and everyone can be overwhelmed by the din. A sensitive child may feel like the teacher yelled at the class when she was simply trying to be heard.

Here are some ways to manage noise level in the classroom:

- Teachers can turn lights on and off or play a certain piece of music to get students' attention rather than raising their own voices.

- If chairs make abrasive scraping noises when moved on the bare floor, add tennis balls with an X-shaped cut in to the chair feet. You can get used tennis balls from the gym or a tennis school or buy pre-cut Chair Sox online and from stores like Lakeshore Learning.

- To help students concentrate and block out the distracting sound of scratching pencils, sniffles, coughs, and talking, it helps to have white noise to level out some of these sounds. Fish tanks, white noise machines, white or pink noise CDs, or a White Noise iPhone app can all help.

- Music played at low volume may help some students focus, but may defocus others. Use music judiciously in the classroom. While Mozart or Chopin are classic choices for concentration, consider other music such as ambient music by Brian Eno or nature-based music such as Gentle Sounds (vitallinks.com). Remember that what makes YOU or the teacher relax may not be relaxing for a student who may actually need quiet in order to focus.

- Another option is to allow students who are organized by music listen to the music that suits them best over headphones during reading, drawing, and other focus times. Help students figure out when they benefit from music and when silence is, in fact, golden.

- Allow students to wear ear protection such as headphones for times when they need quiet.

• The Yacker Tracker can help students gain insight into just how noisy they are as a group. Designed to look like a traffic light, the Yacker Tracker monitors noise levels in the classroom (or other room in the school) and alerts students when noise has reached an unacceptable level set by the teacher (from yackertracker.com and many therapy catalogs).

Visual Overloading

Today's classroom teachers typically do not have the choice to decorate their rooms as they see fit to meet their students' learning needs. Instead, they may be told how to decorate their walls to meet district requirements. As an unfortunate result, classroom walls are now packed with visuals some students find overwhelming.

Teachers can provide some respite for sensitive children by taking these steps:

• Avoid unnecessary decorations on walls.

• If a student is distracted by mandatory wall decorations, cover them with plain paper during key times such as essential lectures, in-class essays, and so on.

• Allow students to wear caps in class if disturbed by overhead lighting (check school policy).

• Use a small area of the room as a cozy nook with reduced visuals and reduced lighting.

• Provide a clear work surface, that is, no unnecessary papers or books on the child's desk.

• Remind parents to provide a quiet, nondistracting, nicely lit workspace at home for homework and other activities that require the child to focus.

• Incorporate individual study carrels to reduce distraction and boost concentration.

• Allow students to take tests and write in-class essays in a separate location (this often needs to be on the IEP or 504 Plan).

• Double-check that all written materials are printed clearly and cleanly since, over time, copies of copies of copies of handouts and worksheets become increasingly hard to read.

- Simplify worksheets if they are overcrowded, enlarging type size as needed.

- Experiment with colored overlays and colored papers to see if reducing the contrast between the paper and the black type will be more visually soothing to students.

Reading Time

A significant number of students with attention and sensory problems have undiagnosed poor visual acuity and/or visual processing problems. Signs to look for include squinting, rubbing eyes, blinking, covering one eye, tilting the head when looking at a book or other close-up object, or frequent complaints of headache, tiredness, or boredom when reading.

A thorough vision examination from a qualified vision care provider should be conducted if there is any concern about the child's visual system and especially if the child is struggling with reading. This should be done by either a developmental optometrist (also called a behavioral optometrist) or a pediatric ophthalmologist who specializes in the development of children's functional vision opposed to just diseases and surgery of the eyes. A vision screening by a parent volunteer, school nurse, or even a pediatrician is not a comprehensive vision examination.

Of course, students with visual acuity problems should wear reading glasses if they have been prescribed. Eyeglasses may also be prescribed to relax the eye muscles if the child struggles with convergence insufficiency or convergence excess (see Chapter 3). The teacher may need to reinforce wearing of the eyeglasses as recommended and may need to frequently check that the eyeglass lenses are clean and smudge free.

Good, comfortable lighting is obviously quite important whether a student is just learning to read or poring over texts for hours. Even with good visual acuity, some visually sensitive students may struggle with contrast sensitivity. Their eyes and brains can't deal with the sharp contrast between the white paper and the black typeface. Some students will benefit from using colored acetate overlays that reduce the contrast and relax the eye, empowering the student to read better.

While children are expected to be able to visually scan the written page easily from left to right, word by word, and then shift down to the leftmost side of the next line, others need some support to do so. For these readers, it should be okay to use a finger to keep track of each word. For others, a piece of plain cardboard or a ruler placed over upcoming lines of print can help a child scan efficiently across a line of print and eliminate the visual distraction of other lines of type. If need be, the student can use an appropriately sized typoscope that covers all but a few words at a time. Typoscopes can be purchased from therapy catalogs and elsewhere online or cut carefully to size out of thick card stock or cardboard.

Teaching a student to use highlighter markers or strips (from therapy catalogs and online from places like enasco.com) helps draw visual attention to the most salient points in written materials. This enhances visual attention and makes reviewing written material for tests easier.

Children who struggle with reading often become self-conscious when reading out loud in the classroom. Since they may still need to practice reading aloud, it helps to be assured that the audience is non-judgmental. The Tail Waggin' Tutors reading program from Therapy Dogs International (tdi-dog.org) may be an excellent solution. Spending time with a gentle therapy "literacy dog"—petting and reading to him—makes it pleasurable and fun while building self-esteem and motivating a student to read without the fear of being judged by other people.

Writing Time

Competent handwriting is an essential skill students must achieve to satisfy basic scholastic demands in elementary school (Volman, van Schendel, & Jongmans, 2006). A whopping 30 percent of students' time revolves around fine motor activities, with handwriting as the single most common task (McHale & Cermak, 1992). Thus, proficiency in handwriting is an important key to school success. Handwriting proficiency is assessed in terms of both legibility and speed of production.

Anywhere from 5 percent to over one-quarter of students demonstrate handwriting difficulties (Hamstra-Bletz & Blote, 1990). When you analyze the components of handwriting, it's easy to see why so many students struggle with learning to write, getting their thoughts written on paper, and taking notes. A continuous interaction between motor, perceptual, language, and sensory components makes this a very complex task, which some students struggle to master despite their best efforts, resulting in a diagnosis of dysgraphia.

To handwrite optimally, students require the following:

- Trunk, shoulder, and upper arm muscle tone, strength, and stability that keep the body secure while brain and hands are busy.

- Visual acuity and ocular-motor skills that enable eyes to see clearly, read across lines of print, and refocus from near to far and back when taking notes.

- Visual perception and visual memory skills to perceive and reproduce horizontal, vertical, diagonal, and circular forms in accurate relationship to each other in space.

- Fine motor dexterity and ability to use proprioceptive feedback from finger joints and muscles to grade muscle force and joint pressure.

- Ability to integrate visual skills with motor skills as the writer uses vision to guide hand movements to form letters precisely and legibly.

- Cognitive skills such as deciding what to write, organizing thoughts, and then sustaining focus until the writing task is complete.

- Phonemic awareness, defined as hearing, identifying, and manipulating small, individual sounds called phonemes in spoken words, essential to reproducing words and sentences in written form.

Sensory processing difficulties make handwriting even more challenging. In particular, these may include the following:

- Visual sensitivity to light, especially to glare, downcast lighting, and fluorescents.

- Visual overloading when lined paper is confusing or poorly printed, a worksheet is too crowded, or contrast sensitivity makes black letters on white paper appear to jiggle.

- Tactile sensitivity to paper, writing tool, and writing surface.
- Auditory sensitivity to the teacher's voice, sounds of other students writing, and ambient noise.

The following are some key ways to help.

Prepare Bodies and Brains to Write

In addition to the movement activities described earlier in this chapter, teachers can get students of any age ready to write by having them drink some water, eat something crunchy, chew gum, and engage in upper body warm-ups such as these:

- Shoulder shrugs: Standing tall, pull your shoulders up to your ears and then push them all the way down and back. Do this five times and keep them down at the end.
- Painting circles: Keeping shoulders down, bring arms straight out to the sides. Imagine you are holding two paintbrushes with your favorite color paint, and paint circles on both sides of the room. Do this 5–10 times circling clockwise, and then 5–10 times circling counterclockwise (5 times for young children, 10 times for older students).
- Karate finger flicks: to strengthen hands and arms and build body awareness, hold arms straight out, palms down. Alternate between making a fist and fully extending fingers quickly 10 times. Then turn palms upward and repeat 10 times. Great as a prewriting activity.
- Pop strips of bubble wrap with fingertips or tape large pieces to the wall and have students pop bubbles by pushing against them. Kids can also pop bubbles by stomping bubble wrap on the floor.
- Model Magic clay, Play-Doh with a Fun Factory, and Alex's Clay Pictures are great for giving tactile and proprioceptive input to fingers, wrists, and arms for younger children. Sculpey, Theraputty, Crazy Aaron's Thinking Putty, and Putty Elements offer greater resistance and sensory input suitable for older students.
- Pop beads and snap-together toys are wonderful. Recommendations include Parents brand pop beads, Tricky Tree and bear/star/heart beads (pfot.com), textured pop beads (thepencilgrip.com), and activities for older students such as pop bead DNA (epicofevolution.com).

- Other great toys that provide good motor preparation include Zoomball and Tricky Tree (pfot.com); Lite Brite; Perler fuse beads and Fun Fusion beads (with tweezers for greater challenge); ZooSticks, FishSticks, and other connected tongs to pick up small items including snacks; dot-to-dots; Tic Tac Toe and Connect Four (teaches diagonals); and mazes, lacing cards, stringing beads, Don't Break the Ice, Alex's My Tissue Art, Color by Number (markers or colored pencils), Shrinky Dinks, Kumon books for scissor skills, and many others.

Take a Multisensory Approach

Most students pick up handwriting skills with a little practice with crayons, markers, pencils, and paper. Other children benefit from a multisensory approach and much more practice. Rolling out play dough into "snakes" to form letter shapes, painting letters, writing them with a finger in pudding, tracing them on a carpet square, or writing them with a stick in mud are all fun, tactile ways to learn letter formation.

Structured handwriting programs can make a huge difference. One of the best and most popular ones is called Handwriting Without Tears (HWTears.com). This easy-to-learn curriculum includes hands-on activities and engaging lessons for pre-K through fifth grade, and has been adopted by an increasing number of school systems. The program starts with songs and wood shapes to form letters without requiring advanced fine motor skills, progresses to writing simplified, vertically oriented letters with chalk, and then introduces pencils with engaging workbooks for each skill level.

Handwriting Boosters

There are several modifications to the handwriting experience that can help, ranging from adapted writing tools to writing surfaces. Of course, children who are unable to produce handwritten work are entitled by IDEA to use assistive technology.

Pencil Grasp Development

Occupational therapists are frequently consulted to remediate the way students hold their pencils. A "mature" pencil grasp is one in which just the fingers and wrist move instead of the entire arm and shoulder. This empowers students to make finely controlled movements of the pencil in order to write and draw.

The palm of the hand is perfect for holding something spherical like a ball. While it's typical for a 12–18-month-old child to use a primitive, fisted palm-based grasp, often with a bent wrist, it's not an acceptable way for a school-age child to hold a writing tool.

The next step in grasp development is usually the pronated grasp seen in toddlers ages 2–3. Here the child holds crayons with straight fingers with the wrist facing downward toward the paper. The child then moves the entire arm to color or scribble. This immature grasp pattern will not work well for the school-age child.

After age 3, the child learns to slightly flex his fingers, typically four fingers, to hold the pencil with the arm still moving. This is called the static quadrupod grasp. Between ages 3½ and 4, the child ideally learns to use just three fingers in a static tripod grasp. In both grasp patterns, the "web space" between the thumb and the index finger is partially or completely closed. Because the entire arm moves rather than the finger joints themselves, it is a grasp most suited to scribbles, lines, and curves, and not an appropriate grasp for the finely detailed pencil movements needed to write and draw proficiently.

Next, the child should learn to walk his fingertips down toward the point of his writing tool, opening up that web space between the thumb and the index finger, and learn to move dynamically, that is, just the fingers rather than the entire arm.

Between ages 4½ and 6, the child should ideally develop a dynamic tripod grasp in which she holds the pencil toward the tip with her thumb, index, and middle finger with a rounded web space, using tiny movements of the intrinsic hand muscles to make detailed, small, controlled marks on paper. The positioning allows a child to rest and stabilize her forearm on the tabletop, pinky (ulnar) side down so the fingers can do their work without becoming fatigued. The ability to write longer passages with increasing speed and legibility builds from here.

The dynamic tripod grasp is widely considered the ideal pencil grasp pattern and many therapists and teachers spend a lot of time attempting to teach students this grasp. Some students get stuck at different stages of grasp development for reasons such as weak hand muscles and poor proprioceptive processing in the upper extremity joints, especially within the fingers. At a certain point, parents, therapists, and teachers need to consider whether their endless efforts to change a child's grip are counterproductive, making the student resent everything to do with handwriting.

When you look around at adults who are writing, you will see several grasp patterns being used effectively by your colleague, friends, your own parent, or even the waiter at your favorite restaurant. A dynamic quadrupod grasp in which the pencil is supported by all fingers except the pinky should also be acceptable. Even thumb wrap grasps in which the thumb wraps across the front of the pencil may be end up having to be accepted, although also it does overstretch some hand muscles, resulting in early fatigue. In some Asian countries, holding the pencil between the index and middle fingers with support from beneath by the thumb to control movements is ideal, and in fact this is the most balanced grasp of all from a biomechanical standpoint.

The rule of thumb, so to speak, is whether the muscles of the hand and wrist are in a position so that the person can use her muscles to control the pencil with minute adjustments without fatigue over increasing periods. Meanwhile, there are many modifications and accommodations that can make writing much easier. The earlier these are introduced to the student the better. Preschool is best, though even upper elementary school students may be profoundly grateful when these adjustments are introduced.

Teach Hand and Finger Awareness

It can help to explicitly teach students about parts of their hands and fingers and what they are for. They may need help to discriminate between finger pads and fingertips. You can help them become more aware of how their fingers and hands work by teaching them to massage their forearms, wrists, palms, and fingers, including gently compressing fingertips and nail beds and massaging the web space between the thumb and index finger, which can become tight and painful. They can learn to do this themselves throughout the school day, especially before writing. You can also teach them to rub their hands together briskly to bombard tactile receptors and warm them up. All of these activities are great prior to handwriting work or any fine motor work.

Some kids simply need help learning where to hold the pen or pencil. Some hold the pencil, marker, or crayon too high up toward the eraser tip, making the task of controlling it quite difficult. Children's markers and crayons usually have "holding stripes" so kids can learn where their fingertips should be placed. You can remind them to make a big O with their web space when holding a writing tool.

You can add a thin strip of brightly colored electrical tape from the hardware store in the child's favorite color approximately one inch above the pencil tip and instruct the child to place her fingertips on this tape. Teach her to remove the tape before sharpening the pencil and to replace it in the same spot afterward. This seeming inconvenience will actually reinforce the holding spot.

Molded Pencil Grips

A variety of molded pencil grips can be added to a pencil, colored pencil, or slim marker that can significantly improve grasp as well as sensory comfort for students. It is best to start children using grips as young as possible—preschool or kindergarten—since it gets increasingly difficult to change grasp patterns in an older student. Here are some of the most effective ones:

- The Pencil Grip, an ergonomically designed, molded three-sided grip that provides rubberized cushioning over the hard pencil and provides a side for each finger to promote a tripod grasp. Like most grips, it acts as a cushion for writers who dislike holding a hard pen or pencil. It can be used by righties by placing the thumb on the side marked R or lefties by placing the thumb on the side marked L. It is also available in a jumbo size, which is more suitable for adult-sized hands and those with arthritis.

- The Pencil Grip company's CrossOver Grip uses the same design with the addition of a wing that blocks fingers from crossing over each other. Users place the thumb under one side, and thumb and middle fingers on the other side.

- The Grotto Grip is a harder, less pliable version of the CrossOver with a larger fingertip well below the wing. Many students prefer this harder, less mushy grip to the CrossOver.

- Abilitations Egg Ohs! grips are foam rubber, egg-shaped grips that open up the palm of the child's hand and position fingers in a better way as the child learns to write. These are especially suitable for children with neuromuscular and orthopedic issues.

- The Writing Claw is a fun way to teach students to hold a pencil correctly. The pencil goes through the middle and there are three rubbery cups for the thumb, index, and middle fingertips.

- There are many other grips and pencil adaptations worth asking the OT about, including the Stetro, Start Write Grip, Writing Bird, and HandiWriter, among others.

Tools, Paper, and Surfaces

The pencil or pen itself may also make a difference. Consider these options:

- Chubby pencils and triangular pencils may be easier for a student to hold.

- Weighted pencils and pens add heft and therefore give more proprioceptive feedback to a student with sensory issues. This is also something to try for the student with hand tremors. These are available from the Pencil Grip Company with a built-in pencil grip or may be created for any writing tool by adding specially designed pencil weights available from therapy catalogs and elsewhere.

- Specially designed pens such as the PenAgain and the ergonomic EVO pen entirely change the way the user grasps the pen.

- Vibrating pens wake up hand muscles and attention spans. These include the Squiggle Wiggle Writer, which is lots of fun but difficult to control. The Z-Vibe, well known as an oral motor vibration tool, has a pencil adaptor kit that includes a chewable tip. The similar Tran-Quil pen or pencil set also provides light vibration (therapyshoppe.com).

Using a flat tabletop can make it hard for a student to write comfortably because he may have to crane his neck to see what he is doing or bend his wrist inward (flex) to write. The student may wind up slumped over the desk, finding it hard to stay alert and tuned in.

Using a slant board on a tabletop brings the materials closer to the face so the child does not have to bend over to see. Placing materials at an upward incline pulls the writer's wrist out of a flexed, bent position and into a neutral or slightly extended position that is far more comfortable. Having students stand up and work on a chalkboard, peel-and-stick chalkboard (wallies.com), dry erase board, wall easel, or paper taped to the wall is a fun, engaging whole-body activity that helps student see better, strengthen their bodies, and engage more effectively.

Tabletops are composed of hard, durable material that makes the writing tool slide quickly over the top. You can help a student slow down their writing by adding drag to the surface with a desk pad or polyester nonskid sheeting. Nonskid matting such as Dycem is also great for putting under slant boards, dishes, and other items so they don't move around. If the child is sensitive to light, consider whether light is bouncing off the shiny tabletop into the child's eyes. You can use plastic sheeting or get an old-fashioned desk blotter to eliminate the glare and soften up the writing surface.

Reconsider writing papers as well. Old-fashioned gray or cream paper with solid blue, red, and dotted lines can be confusing for some students, especially those with visual issues. Instead, opt for simple, clean writing papers such as those from Handwriting Without Tears or raised line paper, which uses "fried ink" to raise the lines, providing kids with tactile cues about where letters should go.

All of these grips, pencils, slant boards, desk pads, desk blotters, and other adaptations are available at sensorysmarts.com and most are in therapy catalogs and Web sites such as therapro.com.

Proprioception Tips

Some kids struggle to use sensory feedback from joints, muscles, and connective tissues to grade their force and movement. This makes it hard to exert the appropriate amount of pressure and to form letters legibly.

For kids who tend to press too hard:

- Teach the student to lighten up and practice making very heavy marks versus very light marks to identify something right in the middle.
- Have the child check the back of the paper to see if it is bumpy or ripped.
- Try writing on styrofoam or packing foam and try to not rip through the paper.
- Break crayons and chalk into small pieces.
- Try a mechanical pencil. The lead will break if the person presses too hard, but do watch out for unnecessary frustration.
- Use a softer pencil.

For kids who tend to press too lightly:

- Engage in hand strengthening work such as using Silly Putty to activate sensory receptors in the joints and muscles before writing.
- Again, teach the child to experiment with heavier versus lighter pressure.
- Use a freshly sharpened pencil.
- Consider an erasable pen.
- Allow the child to color with markers rather than crayons so he gets some satisfaction.

Harnessing Technology

Today's students are more technologically savvy than ever, including preschoolers. Schools and families can leverage this interest to address handwriting issues through various apps and software programs. Some recommended apps are:

- LetterSchool: an amusing and appealing tool for practicing upper- and lowercase letter formations. Can be set in Handwriting Without Tears style (recommended) as well as D'Nealian and Zaner-Bloser styles.
- Touch and Write: a wonderful tool that uses funny writing textures such as ketchup and chocolate frosting for practicing let-

ters, numbers, and high-frequency sight words as well as the child's own name.

- LetterReflex: a hard-working app that helps kids overcome persistent letter reversals through games that help them distinguish between right- and left-sided formations such as d versus b and finger swiping to correct reversed and upside-down letters.

- Dexteria: a fine motor skill app that has kids pinch crabs, tap on colored triangles with particular fingers, and trace over letters.

- Dragon Dictation: converts dictated thoughts into written words with surprising accuracy and lets users copy and paste text into any documents including e-mail. Accessibility options built into computers such as the iPad and Mac can be set to read text out loud to help users hear what needs to be edited. They are good choices for students and adults with dysgraphia and dyslexia who speak articulately but have trouble writing and editing.

- Other fun word apps include Word Builder, Scramble With Friends, Words with Friends, Jumbline, and Wurdle.

Check out otswithapps.com for a wide variety of applications including apps for reading, text-to-speech, spell checking, and adapting worksheets for use on iPads as well as other mobile devices such as Android. Momswithapps.com is another good resource.

Getting Thoughts on Paper

It is important to differentiate between handwriting that is slow due to difficulties with physical production and that which is slow due to difficulties with the development and organization of thought.

While young writers in the early grades write slowly as they produce individual letter strokes, students in older grades should be able to write more rapidly and automatically, directing their attention and focus to expressing concepts and ideas. While children should always be encouraged to improve their handwriting, most studies show that handwriting development plateaus by third grade (Hamstra-Bletz & Blote, 1990) or at the very latest sixth grade as writers develop a personalized writing style (Graham, Berninger, Weintraub, & Schafer, 1998).

When ability to produce written work interferes with written communication, it's time to consider ways to facilitate getting those ideas on paper. An assistive technology evaluation that assesses speed and legibility of handwritten work versus typing speed and accuracy will help determine whether keyboarding and other assistive devices should be introduced and to what extent technology should be incorporated into daily schoolwork.

It is essential that students with graphomotor challenges learn to keyboard early. Students with sensory issues may do best with a typing tutorial program that does not have distracting music and colorful graphics and games. One such program is UltraKey (downloadable from bytesoflearning.com). Of course, if graphics and games will help to motivate the student, there are many programs worth investigating.

More and more schools have Macs and other computers in the classroom and are encouraging students to use laptops and other devices for schoolwork. Today's laptop computers and portable keyboards such as the AlphaSmart NEO or Dana (from neo-direct.com) are lightweight and portable, but it is harder to sit erect when using them because the child must direct her gaze downward instead of at eye level as with a desktop computer. If students complain of headaches or neck pain, this is a key area to consider.

Taking notes in class can be profoundly difficult for many students. Here are a few tips for dealing with this:

- The teacher should provide a set of written notes for students.
- Teach the student not to write every word the teacher says. Practice listening for keywords as well as using abbreviations and outlining lectures.
- The student can record the lecture with a SmartPen, a special pen that has a built-in recorder and uses special paper on which the student can outline the lecture. When reviewing class notes, the student touches the pen to sections of the handwritten notes to have the pen play back that part of the lecture.

Lunchtime

Eating in the school cafeteria can be very challenging for children given the oftentimes unappetizing industrial food, unpleasant food aromas and smells of powerful cleaning products such as ammonia-based cleansers, boisterous students talking and walking around, uncomfortable benches and tables that may not suit the child's size, fluorescent lighting, and of course the cavernous open space that echoes with the noise of kids and clatter of trays, cutlery, and so on. Balancing food on a tray while walking, using poorly finished and thus scratchy plastic utensils and dishware, all while trying to socialize may all be a bit or a lot too much for a sensitive child. The following are some lunchtime strategies.

Deal With Smell and Taste Issues

Have the parents send in well-tolerated food from home. Encourage the student to sniff a preferred essential oil such as sweet orange or vanilla prior to entering the cafeteria so that this is the dominant scent in the child's nostrils. Arrange to have the cafeteria cleaned with nonammonia cleansers at the end of the school day with all the windows open so the room is fully aired out.

Assign a Preferred Seat

A student who is smell sensitive should sit far away from where food is prepared and from garbage and close to a source of ventilation such as an open window. A student who has difficulty balancing her tray should sit close to where the food is served.

Form a Lunch Club

Many students would benefit from avoiding the cafeteria altogether since lunchtime can be such a sensory challenge as well as a social challenge. Some savvy educators and therapists organize special lunch clubs in a classroom, therapy room, or other quiet spot with a small group of children. Children can bring their own lunch, or, in some cases, the teacher or therapist can arrange to have lunch delivered to the room. Lunch clubs can work really well to eliminate the sensory assault of the cafeteria while promoting socialization and even some extra academic support. This may need to be added to the Individualized Education Program (IEP).

Test Time

Sensory issues can interfere with the ability to take tests to the best of a student's ability because of distractions from the sound and smell of classmates, the overhead lighting, and so on. Test accommodations are easily implemented but may need to be formally added to the student's IEP. Common test accommodations include these:

- Taking the test in a separate location such as a quiet, pleasantly lit room. This lets a sensitive child demonstrate what she knows without having to deal with sensory distractions.
- Extended time for children who take longer to process information or who write slowly.
- Answers recorded in a variety of ways, such as typing into a computer or dictating to someone (a scribe).
- Allowing a student to chew gum or drink water during the test.
- Allowing the student to take a brief movement break during the test.

Fire Drills

Typical high-pitched fire alarms ringing at ear-splitting volume can be painful and traumatic for sensitive students. A student may take hours, days, or even weeks to recuperate from the fear and pain of a fire drill and become anxious in anticipation of the next one. Alarm systems with strobes can pack a double whammy for visually sensitive kids and those prone to seizures.

Obviously all local fire ordinances must be strictly followed. However, the school system does have a choice about which fire alarm system to use and when and how to conduct fire drills. More modern systems can be set to a safe but lower volume with selectable, less jarring sirens. Even with a tight budget, this may be a wise investment if fire alarms interfere with students' ability to comfortably participate at school.

Fire drills are intended to teach safe behavior in the unlikely event of an actual fire. The potential of a fire is scary enough for many students. The element of surprise may reduce their ability to practice necessary behaviors such as staying calm and following directions. Fire drills do not have to be unannounced interruptions. They can be scheduled at a time that works best. For example, a fire drill can be conducted five minutes before recess so that students only have to walk up and down the stairs once in midafternoon, for example.

In fact, fire drills are intended to help students practice how they will react if there ever is an actual fire. An announced drill will allow them to grab a coat, handbag, or ear protection. Students should have the right to wear noise-reducing earplugs, headphones, or earmuffs in the event of a fire drill. They will still be able to hear the siren and directions.

If fire drills cause severe, prolonged distress not prevented by ear protection and other measures, a student should be warned in advance of fire drills and allowed to leave the building a few minutes before the scheduled drill. This should be added to the IEP and a staff member assigned along with a backup person.

Gym and Recess

Gym and recess should be times when students can play, blow off excess energy, get physically fit, and feel great. Unfortunately, this is not the case for some students.

Gym Class

General education gym classes, whether held in a dedicated gymnasium or in the school cafeteria, tend to be held in large, brightly lit rooms that lack sound-absorbing materials. This can result in strong echoes as the sound of voices, whistles, balls, and other gym equipment bounce around the room. The sensory experience is usually magnified and sometimes made intolerable by a gym teacher who blows a shrill whistle to get attention. All too often, students are directed to

enter the room quietly and sit while the gym teacher explains the day's
gym activity. Students can benefit from these strategies:

- Give students five minutes to move before asking them to sit down
  and be quiet.
- In elementary school, have the gym teacher come to the classroom
  to discuss the day's activity and then lead the class to the gym.
- Add sound-absorbing mats to the room.
- Eliminate the gym whistle, opting instead to turn the light switch
  on and off if student attention is required.
- Allow sensitive students to work in a smaller group if possible.
- Consider whether the student is eligible for Adaptive Physical
  Education class, which is mandated under IDEA for students with
  disabilities. Such classes also tend to be held in large rooms but
  typically they are at least conducted in smaller groups and led by
  a specialist in physical fitness for kids with special needs.

Recess

Recess is the highlight of the school day for many students, but it
can be a tense time for those with sensory processing issues.

Kids who are sensory seekers may look forward to recess all morning, just waiting for a chance to obtain the input their bodies need.
This is the perfect time for them to get vestibular input through running, swinging, spinning, climbing, hanging upside down, playing in
the sandbox, and so on. Some sensory-seeking kids become disorganized in their behavior because of their intense craving for input. It
will help them to make a plan before going out and to practice safe,
appropriate behaviors. For example, the child who tends to run to a
desired piece of playground equipment, knocking over classmates in
his path, may work with a teacher or therapist to practice navigating
obstacle courses, including moving people. Risk takers may need to
be reminded of safety rules to avoid impulsive sensory-seeking behaviors like jumping off the top of the monkey bars.

Kids who tend to get overloaded are especially at risk at recess
because classmates are speaking loudly, running haphazardly, and

there is sound and movement everywhere. The oversensitive student may retreat to a corner and avoid participating in playground activities. Strategies that may help this student:

- Wear ear protection such as noise-canceling headphones that dampen sound.
- Wear sunglasses or a wide-brimmed cap outside.
- Play with a small group of students, for example, hitting a tennis ball against a wall, completing an obstacle course, using sidewalk chalk, playing hopscotch, shooting hoops and so on.
- Have recess time in a smaller, more contained space such as an alcove with supervision for safety.
- Have occupational or physical therapy sessions scheduled on the playground at this time.

Exercise is essential to students' well-being, especially for those who crave movement such as kids with ADHD (Hallowell & Ratey, 2005). Some schools consider recess a reward for good work in class and will withhold recess as a way to discipline a child who has misbehaved or to make up missed schoolwork. This is counterproductive for two main reasons:

- First, repeated studies have determined that having a recess period results in behavioral improvements. For example, a study found that having more than one recess period of at least 15 minutes a day was associated with improved classroom behavior (Barros, Silver, & Stein, 2009). By providing students with a change of pace and release of energy, recess enables students to be less fidgety and more attentive to academic tasks, according to the National Association of Early Childhood Specialists (2002). Further, study after study shows that physical fitness in school leads to better grades (Pontifex, Saliba, Raine, Picchietti, & Hillman, 2012).
- Second, for students who have difficulty during recess, misbehaving is an excellent way to get out of it. For example, if a student dislikes bright light, noisy kids, and group games, staying indoors and sitting quietly with a book while classmates go out would be quite appealing and easily achieved if it is school policy to discipline by keeping students indoors during recess.

Rather than depriving students of recess, it's essential to determine the underlying causes of misbehavior. In other words, always attempt to treat the root cause rather than the symptoms. Does the child have a learning difference that makes it hard for him to follow along in class? Is anything going on that is causing emotional stress? Does he need a short movement break to stay focused? Is he avoiding sensory overload during outdoor time? Is recess time too unstructured and therefore overwhelming for a student?

If it is clear that this student needs recess to stay on an even keel, parents can get a pediatrician's note stating that the child must have a recess period every day. Mandatory recess can then be written into the child's IEP.

Transitions Between Activities and Classes

Some students have trouble with transitions between classes or activities. It may be that the student has trouble with changes—from indoors to outdoors, being in a crowded hallway between classes, or simply changing mind-set. Such transitions are prime time for sensory overload. Here are a few tips:

- Provide verbal notice about upcoming transitions. Use a visual timer if it helps. Try playing soft music to help kids recognize that something is about to change and they need to be ready to refocus their attention. Whether a young child is busy building a castle with Duplo blocks or reading a chapter book, hearing this music, first at a very soft volume and then a bit louder, is an excellent cue. Some teachers gently play a tambourine or triangle.

- Keep lights low during transitions in and out of the classroom or between activities to keep noise volume down. Encourage children to whisper as they get ready to enter the hallway.

- If children are required to stand in line and have difficulty doing so, provide an actual line taped onto the floor. Allow the child who avoids casual touch to stand at the end of the line or to engage in a special task during line-up.

- Allow older, more independent students to be first to leave the room in order to get to the next class before the hallway is jam-packed with students. Or allow the student to be a few moments late without penalty. Keep in mind, however, that being first in the classroom is less noticeable and taunt-worthy than always being late.

Climbing stairs is a great sensory diet activity for students. This intense "heavy work" activates the deep, large muscles of the body and provides tons of proprioceptive input, giving students and teachers short, healthy workouts throughout the school day.

However, going up and down stairs can be tricky for some kids due to any combination of neuromuscular and sensory processing challenges. They may feel crowded in by other students and may refuse to climb stairs or may push others out of the way in self-protection. If possible, the student should be escorted up and down stairs discreetly, either at the end of the line or possibly before or after other children have descended.

Ascending stairs requires good muscle strength, particularly in the legs, as well as endurance and lung power. A student with poor body awareness and/or low muscle tone who struggles with an under-aroused nervous system may climb stairs slowly because it is such hard work. This student should certainly work with a PT on strengthening and safe stair climbing. If safety or physical strength and endurance are an issue and there are several flights to climb several times a day, the student should be entitled to use the elevator if one is available. This will need to be added to the IEP.

Descending stairs also requires good muscle control and body awareness, with a strong visual component. If visual skills are lacking, a child may have perfectly good strength and physical coordination but still be extremely cautious about going down a flight of stairs because it feels like he is stepping out into space. A child who has difficulties with depth perception cannot accurately perceive where the next step is and may feel like going downstairs is more an act of faith than anything else.

Double-check that all stairs are well illuminated with light that is not glaring. The edges of each step should be clearly demarcated. Reflective stair tape (available at many hardware stores or online from sites such as seton.com) is a quick fix but may peel off or wear poorly, especially on outdoor stairs. Reflective paint, such as that used on roads and on some playgrounds, contains tiny glass beads that reflect light and offers a more permanent, safer stair edge marker. Again, if safety is an issue, use of an elevator should be considered and added to the IEP.

Special Class Considerations

Art Class

Art projects in the student's own classroom or in a separate art room can pose distinct and significant sensory challenges. Art media such as paint, markers, glue, and clay typically have a strong smell that is intolerable for some students. Tactile exploration may be delightful for sensory seekers and completely noxious for others. The goal here is participation, and sensory issues should not prevent that.

Students should be allowed to wear soft, oversized shirts from home instead of smocks that may be unbearable because of the fabric texture or scratchy neck closures.

If a student refuses to get messy, offer gloves and a long-handled paintbrush or glue sticks instead of liquid glue. Sometimes having a damp cloth nearby for wiping hands can make all the difference. Once children find pleasure in what they are doing, they are usually more willing to deal with the sensory aspects.

Special attention should be paid to having good ventilation during art projects, opening a window or using a fan if necessary. It is essential that a teacher avoid invalidating a sensitive student by saying, "It doesn't smell." It does. Everything smells like something. Even if the label states the item is certified nontoxic, it may still be toxic to a student's sensitive nervous system. If the student cannot tolerate the smell of regular markers or tempera paint, try alternatives such as Mr. Sketch scented markers or liquid watercolor paint. Colored pencils and crayons may be best tolerated. If a student refuses to touch play dough or regular clay, try fruit-scented Lakeshore dough, unscented gluten-free Wonder Dough, or low-residue Crayola Model Magic.

Older kids might enjoy using Sculpey, which hardens when baked to make beads and other objects.

Science Class

In science classes, smell can be a challenge since stinky chemicals may be used in the room. Remember that even if these smelly materials are not used during the child's own science period, the hyper-sensitive smeller will still have to contend with them in the air. All chemicals and smelly materials should be stored as far away as possible, preferably in a room not used by students. The smell-sensitive student can be given a preferred essential oil to sniff prior to science and art classes to preempt intolerable odors.

Many science classes have students sit on high stools to enable them to peer more easily into microscopes, pour with beakers, and so on. This may be physically challenging for students with poor postural control and body awareness. These students will benefit from height-adjustable stools that have back support (such as those available at k-log.com).

Assemblies

Any large gathering of students is ripe for discomfort for an auditory-sensitive student. The student should be entitled to wear ear protection to any school assembly and should be seated at the end of the row near an exit so he can take a break if needed without disturbing classmates. Students should be allowed to bring seat cushions and hand fidgets if this helps them to participate in this school activity.

Music Class

For the auditory-defensive student, music class can be pure cacophony. The student should be allowed to wear noise-canceling headphones and given preferential seating farthest away from loud instruments. If the din is intolerable, investigate whether requirements can be met through alternative arrangements such as one-on-one music lessons.

End of the School Day

Even for kids who are more than ready to finish their school day, dismissal may be a stressful transition. For the student who has trouble getting organized, whether due to sensory distractions, attention challenges, or executive function deficits, an aide or teacher can help make sure everything she needs is packed in her book bag, and double-check that she has written everything legibly in an assignment notebook. If transporting books necessary for homework is too difficult for this student, a second set of books should be available to keep at home.

Again, consider whether this student should be allowed to leave at a staggered time—either a few minutes ahead of other students or after most others have left.

After-school Activities

Weigh after-school activities carefully. Many kids with sensory issues will be thrilled to let off some steam in an after-school Tae Kwon Do or dance class and have plenty of energy left for doing homework afterward. Others may love the quiet discipline of an after-school chess club or drawing lessons.

Other kids require some down time after school. Some students expend a lot of emotional and physical energy keeping it together all day at school and are quite exhausted when school lets out. For these kids, nothing may be more beneficial than to spend some time in a relaxing place—whether it's a pretty park looking at ducks or a quiet bedroom with toys and books. It is very important to assess whether a student requires down time or active time after school.

For students with parents who are still at work during after-school hours, it may not be possible for the child to go home if no home-based child care is available. In such situations, the student may have to attend an after-school program. If so, care should be taken to best match the child's sensory needs with the program activities. It should be okay for the child who needs to regroup for a while to do so.

Active participation in an intolerable group activity in this optional rather than mandatory program should not be strictly demanded. If the child needs to take 20 minutes with a book or to listen to favorite music over headphones before playing a game with classmates or doing her homework, this should be acceptable and clearly communicated to the people running the after-school activity.

For a student who is picked up by a parent or other caregiver after school, discuss whether this student needs down time or active time. A parent may not recognize how hard it is for a child to run a series of errands after school and then to sit down and do homework. A child may first need low-stimulation time alone in a quiet, dimly lit room with cozy clothing and furniture, or soothing, reorganizing input such as lots of hugs or a deep pressure massage, or intense movement such as taking a bike ride, swimming, a trip to the playground, or rough-and-tumble play.

Parents may find that even if it is inconvenient, taking time to meet their child's sensory needs first before running any necessary errands or starting homework winds up saving time in dealing with an upset, overloaded child.

Getting Teachers and Parents on Board

Many teachers and school administrators already know about sensory problems. They understand that a child may need a hand fidget in order to self-regulate and attend at circle time, do 20 jumping jacks or climb a few flights of stairs before sitting down to work on handwriting, or wear earplugs during recess and assemblies to protect from unbearable noise.

At the same time, many teachers and school staff haven't heard about SPD or simply don't "believe" in it. Happily, more and more regular and special education teachers, therapists, and behaviorists are following a collaborative model. After all, they all have the same goal—to empower the student to access the educational curriculum to the greatest extent possible. The behaviorist working with a child who acts out in the lunchroom needs to understand auditory hypersensitivity. The speech therapist who is working on expressive and receptive language skills needs to know if the child is distracted by visual input and actually needs to avoid eye contact in order to hear better or needs intense movement to stimulate the vestibular structures connected to the cochlea.

Many parents mistakenly assume that teachers must know about sensory processing issues and how to work around them in school. Or they may keep silent in the hope that this year, the new teacher will not run into the same problems as last year. Or that an older child has overcome his sensory problems entirely because he had such a fabulous, happy summer break. All too often, when these parents learn this is not the case, they may resent having to teach the teachers.

Do counsel parents to speak with teachers and let them know what works for their child. Remind parents that most general education teachers, teaching assistants, and paraprofessionals have received little if any training in atypical development. Special education teachers have received more training, especially in teaching children with disabilities, but again a significant number of these professionals have received little or no information about SPD. This does not entail making unrealistic demands or making a laundry list of things they must do for your child. Truth is, every student is different, and it behooves parents to help the teacher learn how to work best with their particular child. After all, it is the parents who are the ultimate experts.

Taking the time to communicate about the student's unique sensory issues at the beginning of the school year will save everyone time and headaches. The knowledge and compassion of last year's teacher unfortunately may not travel to next year's classroom. Each new school year will bring a new cast of players into the child's life, who will again need to gain insight into and compassion for all of their students—especially those with sensory processing challenges. Encourage parents to present sensory strategies they know work for their child as a way to make it easier for the teacher within the context of a full and busy classroom.

CHAPTER 8

A Sensory Smart Future

One of the first questions parents ask is whether their child will outgrow sensory processing issues. This can be difficult or even impossible to answer. So much depends on how early on the child's sensory issues are identified, how severe they are, and how intensively they are treated.

Sometimes kids with mild sensory issues are like leaves that have gotten stuck on a rock on their way downriver. They just need a little help getting unstuck so they can travel on their way. Other kids have more significant sensory issues that accompany them in one form or another for their entire lives. Even so, children, teens, and young adults can make enormous strides in taking charge of their sensory experiences and their reactions.

Consider Victoria Sciortino, adopted at 13 months of age from an overseas orphanage (she was the little girl renamed Nina in *Raising a Sensory Smart Child*, but wants to use her real name in this book). When Victoria first arrived in New York City, she was distressed by innocuous sensations such as wind and sun on her skin, and was unable to sit for more than a few minutes before she was again on the go, running on her tiptoes without looking where she was going, racing up and down the hall at home, smashing into classmates at preschool, and then rapidly rocking herself to sleep each night.

Today Victoria is 14 years old. She loves riding horses and has earned several ribbons at equestrian competitions. She skis too. At first she couldn't handle group lessons and completely zoned out. After getting one-on-one training for basic skills, she now benefits from group lessons. She's on the track team, excelling at jumping hurdles and sprinting. Her mom Joanne (Marisa in *Raising a Sensory Smart Child*) says Victoria is the consummate procrastinator but during track season she comes home and gets right to work. All of this vestibular and proprioceptive input calms her brain and body sufficiently and long enough that she can get her homework done. It also helps if she listens to music as she works, rocking to the rhythm of Bob Marley and current pop hits.

While Victoria has learned to obtain the movement her body so clearly craves, she faces lingering sensory challenges. She dislikes washing her face and combing her hair. She will only wear soft

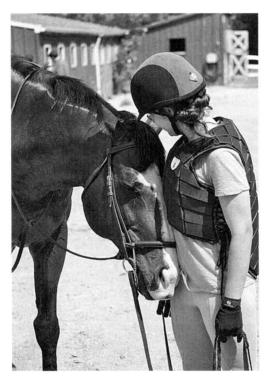

Victoria bonding with Jack before practicing for an upcoming competition. *Photo Courtesy of Joanne Sciortino*

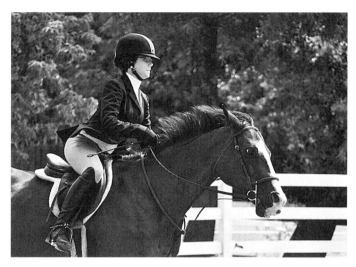

Victoria competing with Jack at a US Equestrian Federation show where she won Reserve Champion (2nd place) for 2'0" jumping. *Photo Courtesy of Joanne Sciortino*

stretchy clothing and absolutely no jeans. She continues to rock back and forth when riding in a car, just as she did as a toddler. She envelops herself in sensory comfort at the end of the day by putting on her one-piece footie pajamas, getting under her microfleece sheets and comforter, and curling up into a tight ball. As she's just beginning to wake up each morning, she rocks to give herself the movement input she has always used to help her feel self-regulated and ready for her day.

Jeremy Sicile-Kira, whom you read about in Chapter 4, uses technology to communicate. He articulated his ongoing sensory challenges:

> When there are bright lights they just hurt. My body can't handle looking someone in the face. When I look at people's faces I need to process what I am seeing. When I process visually I can't use my auditory processing which is the processing type I prefer.
>
> My top need is for an environment that is not too noisy. For example, at the Starbucks near me I sometimes need for it to be quieter. There are a lot of different noises, like the coffee machines and everyone speaking at the same time. My nose can smell every-

thing. The general smell is difficult because I cannot block out the unpleasant ones. The smell of objects and people is distracting and challenging. I can smell the coffee, perfume, deodorant and hand cream of people and it is distracting. The bad smell of smokers' smoke on their clothes is challenging.

My body doesn't like to be touched by random people. I need to prepare for people touching me because it can be very painful. If I know the person usually I can prepare for their touch that I am used to. Strangers are difficult because I don't know how their touch will feel. (Sicile-Kira, personal communication, February 6, 2013)

Now that Jeremy is able to identify exactly what distresses him, he can work on self-regulating in troublesome environments such as the coffee shop and articulating what works best to make him feel better. Jeremy finds that he feels better when:

- Looking at his iPad, which helps him to communicate.
- Looking through a book, such as an art book with beautiful paintings or picture books of animals.
- A support staff member is with him, speaking gently and calmly.
- He goes for a walk, eats, drinks water, wears glasses, or taps on parts of his body.

Jeremy writes:

My top goal is to recognize when it is too noisy before I get overwhelmed. Moving somewhere quieter helps in the beginning before I'm overwhelmed. It helps to set a time limit before we sit down and to make sure there is an exit close by. When it is loud it helps to have my nice book that I carry every day as a transition item on the table. Flipping the pages helps keep me calm.

My second goal is to be able to communicate when I'm overwhelmed. It helps me when I am able to use a "break" card which I keep on my table which I can touch before standing up and going so my support person knows I need to leave. Frankly I always need supports such as my communication partner. It helps when a calm support person is with me. Having a support staff helps because they get everything ready on the table so I can communicate, especially my iPad, my transitional item (a book), and my break card.

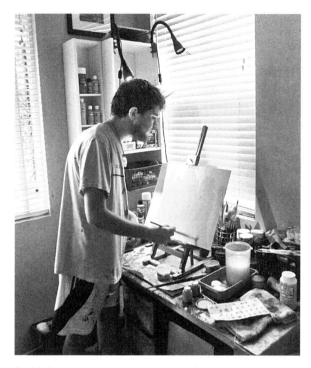

In 2012, Jeremy began painting people using swathes of color. Here he is painting "the aura of Dana with yellow representing her great happiness and brightness" (personal communication, July 13, 2013). Dana is a good friend who recently became engaged. *Photo Courtesy of Chantal Sicile-Kira*

Jeremy has done an enormous amount of work to clarify what sets him off and what helps him stay calm and regulated, and now wishes to help others. He has coauthored a book with his mother called *A Full Life With Autism* and keeps an online blog. He has started to paint, dreaming about and then painting the people he knows and meets. You can see his paintings and follow his blog at Jeremysicile-kira.com. In a March 8, 2013, post, Jeremy wrote, "Trying to be me is hard but I am worth it."

Likewise, helping kids and teens with sensory processing challenges may be hard at times, but it is definitely worth it. Watching sensitive kids grow up into teens and young adults who have mastered their sensory issues is profoundly rewarding.

With time, effort, and patience, your sensitive clients can come to transform their challenges into strengths. A visually hypersensitive client may mature into an artist or architect; a client with auditory issues may become a musician; that picky eater may become a professional chef; and that client with vestibular issues may become an Olympic athlete.

You just never know.

RESOURCES

ONLINE RESOURCES

To help educate parents, schools, and colleagues about sensory processing challenges, consider these free online resources:

> **My child has Sensory Processing Disorder (SPD).**
>
> **My child is out-of-sync right now and needs time to regroup & reorganize.**
>
> Children with SPD misinterpret everyday sensory info, such as touch, sound, smell and movement. They may feel overwhelmed by the world around them or may seek intense sensory experiences.
>
> Visit **www.sensorysmarts.com** and **www.spdfoundation.net** to learn more.
>
> © 2013 sensory street™, inc.
> www.sensorystreet.com

Illustration courtesy of Sensory Street

• sensoryprocessingchallenges.com, this book's Web site.

• Sensorysmarts.com, the Web site for *Raising a Sensory Smart Child*, which contains information for parents, teachers, and others, SPD checklists, where to find an OT, sensory diet activities, videos, and articles.

• SPDFoundation.net offers good information including some of the latest research on SPD.

• Sensory-processing-disorder.com and asensorylife.com.

• Sensorystreet.com, which has great free downloadables including the SPD calling card as well as checklists and handouts such as Melissa Zacherl's *Do You Know Me?* poster available in English, Spanish, and Farsi for parents and in English for teachers.

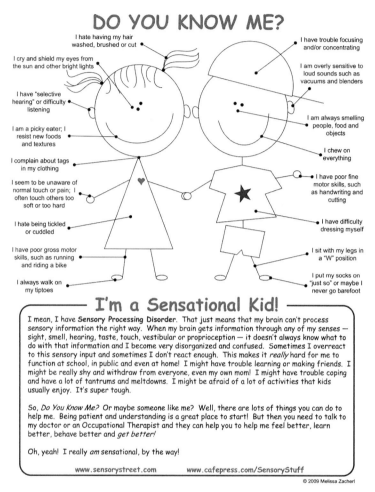

DO YOU KNOW ME?

I hate having my hair washed, brushed or cut

I cry and shield my eyes from the sun and other bright lights

I have "selective hearing" or difficulty listening

I am a picky eater; I resist new foods and textures

I complain about tags in my clothing

I seem to be unaware of normal touch or pain; I often touch others too soft or too hard

I hate being tickled or cuddled

I have poor gross motor skills, such as running and riding a bike

I always walk on my tiptoes

I have trouble focusing and/or concentrating

I am overly sensitive to loud sounds such as vacuums and blenders

I am always smelling people, food and objects

I chew on everything

I have poor fine motor skills, such as handwriting and cutting

I have difficulty dressing myself

I sit with my legs in a "W" position

I put my socks on "just so" or maybe I never go barefoot

I'm a Sensational Kid!

I mean, I have **Sensory Processing Disorder**. That just means that my brain can't process sensory information the right way. When my brain gets information through any of my senses — sight, smell, hearing, taste, touch, vestibular or proprioception — it doesn't always know what to do with that information and I become very disorganized and confused. Sometimes I overreact to this sensory input and sometimes I don't react enough. This makes it *really* hard for me to function at school, in public and even at home! I might have trouble learning or making friends. I might be really shy and withdraw from everyone, even my own mom! I might have trouble coping and have a lot of tantrums and meltdowns. I might be afraid of a lot of activities that kids usually enjoy. It's super tough.

So, *Do You Know Me?* Or maybe someone like me? Well, there are lots of things you can do to help me. Being patient and understanding is a great place to start! But then you need to talk to my doctor or an Occupational Therapist and they can help you to help me feel better, learn better, behave better and *get better!*

Oh, yeah! I really *am* sensational, by the way!

www.sensorystreet.com   www.cafepress.com/SensoryStuff

© 2009 Melissa Zacherl

Illustration courtesy of Melissa Zacherl

RESOURCES FOR SENSORY SMART TOYS AND EQUIPMENT

You may want to start investing in toys and equipment that clients with sensory challenges can use or test out while in your office. You may also want to have catalogs handy for parents, teachers, and others to make it easy to locate recommended items. Some items can be found in brick and mortar stores, on eBay, Amazon, sensorysmarts.com, and elsewhere if you or your clients want to compare prices.

Following are some of the best sensory-specific catalogs. Many companies only show a sampling of what they sell online, so request a print catalog—or several copies for clients—if they have one.

Achievement Products for Special Needs	achievement-products.com
Beyond Play	beyondplay.com
eSpecial Needs (*online only*)	especialneeds.com
Fun and Function	funandfunction.com
Pocket Full of Therapy	pfot.com
Sensory Craver (*online only*)	sensorycraver.com
Sensory Edge (*online only*)	sensoryedge.com
School Specialty's special needs catalog	schoolspecialty.com
Southpaw Enterprises	southpawenterprises.com
The Sensory Spectrum Shop (*online only*)	sensoryspectrumshop.com
Therapro	therapro.com
Therapy Shoppe	therapyshoppe.com

FURTHER READING

Aron, E. (2002). *The highly sensitive child*. New York: Harmony.

Biel, L., & Peske, N. (2009). *Raising a sensory smart child: The definitive handbook for helping your child with sensory processing issues* (rev. ed.). New York: Penguin.

Dagliesh, C.D. (2013). *The sensory child gets organized.* New York: Touchstone.

Dennison, P., & Dennison, G. (1989). *Brain gym: Teacher's edition*. Ventura, CA: Edu Kinesthetics.

Dorfman, K. (2013). *Cure your child with food.* New York: Workman.

Eason, A., & Whitbread, K. (2006). *IEP and inclusion tips for parents and teachers handout version*. Verona, WI: Attainment.

Eide, B., & Eide, F. (2006). *The mislabeled child*. New York: Hyperion.

Ernsberger, L., & Stegen-Hanson, T. (2004). *Just take a bite*. Arlington, TX: Future Horizons.

Grandin, T. (2012). *Different . . . not less: Inspiring stories of achievement and successful employment from adults with autism, Asperger's, and ADHD.* Arlington, TX: Future Horizons.

Grandin, T., & Duffy, K. (2008). *Developing talents: Careers for individuals with asperger syndrome and high-functioning autism.* Overland Park, KS: Autism Asperger.

Hallowell, E. M., & Ratey, J. J. (2005). *Delivered from distraction: Getting the most out of life with attention deficit disorder.* New York: Ballantine.

Heller, S. (2003). *Too loud, too bright, too fast, too tight: What to do if you are sensory defensive in an overstimulating world.* New York: Harper.

Kranowitz, C. (2006). *The out-of-sync child* (rev. ed.). New York: Perigee.

Kuypers, L. (2011). *The zones of regulation.* San Jose, CA: Think Social.

Miller, L. J., & Fuller, D. A. (2007). *Sensational kids.* New York: Perigee.

Potock, M. (2010). *Happy mealtimes with happy kids.* Longmont, CO: My Munch Bug.

Sicile-Kira, C. (2006). *Adolescents on the autism spectrum.* New York: Perigee.

Sicile-Kira, C., & Sicile-Kira, J. (2012). *A full life with autism: From learning to forming relationships to achieving independence.* New York: Palgrave Macmillan.

Siegel, L. (2011). *The complete IEP guide: How to advocate for your special ed child* (7th ed.). Berkeley, CA: Nolo.

Silver, L. B. (1998). *The misunderstood child* (3rd ed.). New York: Three Rivers.

Weissbluth, M. (2005). *Healthy sleep habits, happy child.* New York: Ballatine.

Wrobel, M. (2003). *Taking care of myself: A hygiene, puberty, and personal curriculum for young people with autism.* Arlington, TX: Future Horizons.

REFERENCES

Ahn, R. R., Miller, L. J., Milberger, S., & McIntosh, D. N. (2004). Prevalence of parents' perceptions of sensory processing disorders among kindergarten children. *American Journal of Occupational Therapy, 58*, 287–293.

Allen, A. P., & Smith, A. P. (2011). A review of the evidence that chewing gum affects stress, alertness and cognition. *Journal of Behavioral and Neuroscience Research, 9*, 1, 7–23.

American Academy of Pediatrics. (2012, May 28). Sensory integration therapies for children with developmental and behavioral disorders. *Pediatrics*. doi: 10.1542/peds.2012-0876.

Aspergers Social Stories. (2012). Jeremiah gets a toothache: A Social Story for children with autism (video). Retrieved from http://www.aspergerssocialstories.com/2012/07/jeremiah-gets-toothache-social-story.html

Barros, R., Silver, E., & Stein, R. (2009). School recess and group classroom behavior. *Pediatrics, 123*(2), 431–436.

Basso, M. R. (2001). Neurobiological relationships between ambient lighting and the startle response to acoustic stress in humans. *International Journal of Neuroscience, 110*, 147–157.

Behavior Analyst Certification Board. (2011, September). May BCBAs and BCaBAs implement nonbehavioral interventions? *BACB Online Newsletter*, 1–2..

Bellis, T. J. (2003). *When the brain can't hear: Unraveling the mystery of auditory processing disorder*. New York: Atria.

Ben-Sasson, A., Carter, A. S., & Briggs-Gowan, M. J. (2009). Sensory over-responsivity in elementary school: Prevalence and social-emotional correlates. *Journal of Abnormal Child Psychology, 37*, 705–716.

Bernardi, P., Porta, C., & Sleight, P. (2006). Cardiovascular, cerebrovascular and respiratory changes induced by different types of music in musicians and non-musicians: The importance of silence. *Heart, 92*, 445–452.

Biel, L., & Peske, N. (2009). *Raising a sensory smart child* (rev. ed.). New York: Penguin.

Brown, C., & Dunn, W. (2002). Adolescent/adult sensory profile. Retrieved from Pearson Assessments, pearsonassessments.com

Bunim, J. (2013). Breakthrough study reveals biological basis for sensory processing disorders in kids. Retrieved from UCSF News, http://www.ucsf.edu/news

Cameron, O. G. (2001). Interoception: The inside story—a model for psychosomatic processes. *Psychosomatic Medicine: Journal of Biobehavioral Medicine, 63*, 697–710.

Carruth, B. R., Ziegler, P. J., Gordon, A., & Barr, S. I. (2004, January). Prevalence of picky eaters among infants and toddlers and their caregivers' decisions about offering a new food. *Journal of the American Dietetic Association, 104* (Suppl. 1), 57–64.

Champagne, T. (2006). Creating sensory rooms: Essential enhancements for acute inpatient mental health settings. *Mental Health Special Interest Newsletter, 29*, 1–4.

Champagne, T. (2011). *Sensory modulation and environment: Essential elements of occupation* (3rd ed., rev.). Sydney: Pearson Assessment.

Champagne, T. & Koomar, J. (2011). Expanding the focus: Addressing sensory discrimination concerns in mental health. *Mental Health Special Interest Section Quarterly, 34*(1), 1–4.

Champagne. T., & Stromberg, N. (2004). Sensory approaches in inpatient psychiatric settings: Innovative alternatives to seclusion & restraint. *Journal of Psychosocial Nursing, 42*(9), 1–8.

Chasnoff, I. (2010). *The mystery of risk: Drugs, alcohol, pregnancy and the vulnerable child.* Chicago: NTI Upstream.

Copple, C., & Bredekamp, S. (2009). *Developmentally appropriate practice in early childhood programs, serving children from birth through 8* (rev. ed.). Washington, DC: National Association for the Education of Young Children.

Cytowic, R. E. (1993). *The man who tasted shapes*. New York: Tarcher.

Davies, P. L., & Gavin, W. J. (2007). Validating the diagnosis of sensory processing disorders using EEG technology. *American Journal of Occupational Therapy, 61*, 176–189.

DeGangi, G. (2000). *Pediatric disorders of regulation in affect and behavior*. San Diego, CA: Academic Press.

Dorfman, K. (2013). *Cure your child with food*. New York: Workman.

Dunn, W. (1999). Sensory profile. Retrieved from Pearson Assessments, pearsonassessments.com

Dunn, W. (2002). Infant/toddler sensory profile. Retrieved from Pearson Assessments, pearsonassessments.com

Dunn, W. (2006). Sensory profile school companion. Retrieved from Pearson Assessments, pearsonassessments.com

Eide, B., & Eide, F. (2006). *The mislabeled child*. New York: Hyperion.

Fisher, A. G., & Bundy, A. C. (1989). Vestibular stimulation in the treatment of postural and related disorders. In O. D. Payton, R. P. Di-Fabio, S. V. Paris, E. J. Protas, & A. F. VanSant (Eds.), *Manual of physical therapy techniques* (pp. 239–258). New York: Churchill Livingstone.

Foss-Feig, J. H., Tadin, D., Schauder, K. B., & Cascio, C. J. (2013). A substantial and unexpected enhancement of motion perception in autism. *Journal of Neuroscience, 33*(19), 8243. doi: 10.1523/JNEUROSCI.1608-12.2013.

Gere, D. R., Capps, S. C., Mitchell, D. W., & Grubbs, E. (2009). Sensory sensitivities of gifted children. *American Journal of Occupational Therapy, 63*(3): 288–295.

Graham, S., Berninger, V. W., Weintraub, N., & Schafer, W. (1998). Development of handwriting speed and legibility in grades 1–9. *Journal of Educational Research, 92*, 42–52.

Grandin, T. (2011, November/December). Why do kids with autism stim? *Autism Asperger's Digest*.

Greenspan, S., & Wieder, S. (1997). Developmental patterns and outcomes in infants and children with disorders in relating and communicating. *Journal of Developmental and Learning Disorders, 1*, 87–142.

Hallowell, N., & Ratey, J. (2005). *Delivered from distraction.* New York: Ballantine.

Hamstra-Bletz, L., & Blote, A. W. (1990). Development of handwriting in primary school: A longitudinal study. *Perceptual and Motor Skills, 70*, 759–770.

Herman-Giddens, M. E., Slora, E. J., Wasserman, R. C., Bourdony, C. J., Bhapkar, M. V., Koch, G. G., & Hasemeier, C. M. (1997). Secondary sexual characteristics and menses in young girls seen in office practice: A study from the pediatric research in office settings network. *Pediatrics, 99*, 505–512.

Illi, U. (1994). Balls instead of classroom chairs? *Swiss Journal of Physical Education, 6*, 37–39.

Interdisciplinary Council on Developmental and Learning Disorders (ICDL). (2005). *Diagnostic manual for infancy and early childhood: Mental health, developmental, regulatory-sensory processing, language and learning disorders—ICDL-DMIC* Bethesda, MD: ICDL.

Ishihara, K., Dake, K., Kashihara, T., & Ishihara, S. (2010). An attempt to improve the sitting posture of children in classroom. *Proceedings of International Multiconference of Engineers and Computer Scientists*, Hong Kong, Retrieved from IAENG, http://www.iaeng.org/publication/IMECS2010/IMECS2010_pp1922-1925.pdf.

Jarrow, M. (2010). Occupational therapy and sensory integration. In K. Siri & T. Lyons (Eds.), *Cutting-edge therapies for autism* (pp. 267–276). New York: Skyhorse.

Javitt, D. C. (2009). Sensory processing in schizophrenia: Neither simple nor intact. *Schizophrenia Bulletin, 35*(6), 1059–1064.

King, L. J. (1974). A sensory integrative approach to schizophrenia. *American Journal of Occupational Therapy, 28*(9), 529–537.

Kinnealey, M., & Fuiek, M. (1999). The relationship between sensory over-responsiveness, anxiety, depression and perception of pain in adults. *Occupational Therapy International, 6*, 195–206.

Kuhaneck, H. M., Henry, D. A., & Glennon, T. J. (2007). Sensory processing measure: Main classroom and school environments forms.
Retrieved from Western Psychological Services, wpspublish.com

Kuypers, L. (2011). *The zones of regulation*. San Jose, CA: Think
Social.

Lask, B., Fosson, A., Rolfe, U., & Thomas, S. (1993). Zinc deficiency
and childhood-onset anorexia nervosa. *Journal of Clinical Psychiatry, 54*(2), 63–66.

Leekam, S. R., Nieto, C., Libby, S. J., Wing, L., & Gould, J. (2007).
Describing the sensory abnormalities of children and adults with
autism. *Journal of Autism and Developmental Disorders, 37*,
894–910.

Marco, E. J., Hinkley, L. B., Hill, S. S., & Nagarajan, S. S. (2011). Sensory processing in autism: A review of neurophysiologic findings.
Pediatric Research, 69, 48–54.

Martel, L. D. (2003, July 24). Light: An element in the ergonomics of
learning. *National Academy of Integrative Learning.*

Massachusetts Department of Mental Health. (2007). *Developing
positive cultures of care: Resource guide.* Retrieved from www.
mass.gov/eohhs/docs/dmh/rsri/restraint-resources.pdf

May-Benson, T., & Koomar, J. A. (2007). Identifying gravitational
insecurity in children: A pilot study. *American Journal of Occupational Therapy, 61*(2), 142–147.

McHale, K., & Cermak, S. (1992). Fine motor activities in elementary
school: Preliminary findings and provisional implications for children with fine motor problems. *American Journal of Occupation
Therapy, 46*(10), 898–903.

McIntosh, D. N., Miller, L. J., Shya, V., & Hagerman, R. J. (1999). Sen-
sory-modulation disruption, electrodermal responses, and functional behaviors. *Developmental Medical and Child Neurology,
41*, 608–615.

Miller, L. J., Anzalone, M. E., Lane, S. J., Cermak, S. A., & Osten, E.
T. (2007). Concept evolution in sensory integration: A proposed
nosology for diagnosis. *American Journal of Occupational Therapy, 61*, 135–140.

Miller, L. J., Nielson, D., & Schoen, S. (2012). Attention deficit hyperactivity disorder and sensory modulation disorder: A comparison of behavior and physiology. *Research in Developmental Disabilities, 33*, 804–818.

Miller, L. J., Reisman, J., McIntosh, D. N., & Simon, J. (2001). An ecological model of sensory modulation: Performance of children with fragile X syndrome, autism, attention-deficit hyperactivity disorder and sensory modulation dysfunction. In S. Smith-Roley, E. Imperatore-Blanche, & R. C. Schaaf (Eds.), *Understanding the nature of sensory integration with diverse populations* (pp. 57–88). San Antonio, TX: Therapy Skill Builders.

National Association of Early Childhood Specialists in State Departments of Education. (2002). *Recess and the importance of play: A position statement on young children and recess.* Urbana, IL: National Association of Early Childhood Specialists in State Departments of Education. Retrieved from http://www.eric.ed.gov/PDFS/ED463047.pdf

One Place for Special Needs. (2013). Getting an EEG test—social story. Retrieved from http://www.oneplaceforspecialneeds.com/main/library_eeg_test.html

Owen, J. P., Marco, E. J., Desai, S., Fourie, E. Harris, J., Hill, S. S., Arnett, A. B., & Mukherjee, P. (2013). Abnormal white matter microstructure in children with sensory processing disorders. *Neuroimage: Clinical.* doi:/10.1016/j.nicl.2013.06.009.

Paradiz, V. (2009). *The integrated self-advocacy ISA curriculum.* Shawnee Mission, KS: Autism Asperger.

Parham, D. L., & Ecker, C. (2007). Sensory processing measure: Home form. Retrieved from Western Psychological Services, wpspublish.com

Pfeiffer, B., Henry, A., Miller, S., & Witherell, S. (2008). The effectiveness of Disc 'O' Sit cushions on attention to task in second-grade students with attention difficulties. *American Journal of Occupational Therapy, 62*, 274–281.

Pontifex, M. B., Saliba, B. J., Raine, L. B., Picchietti, D. L., & Hillman, C. H. (2012). Exercise improves behavioral, neurocognitive, and scholastic performance in children with ADHD. *Journal of Pediatrics, 162*, 543–551.

Rapoport, J., & Ismond, D. (1996). *DSM-IV training guide for diagnosis of childhood disorders*. New York: Brunner-Routledge.

Ray, T. C., King, L. J., & Grandin, T. (1988). The effectiveness of self-initiated vestibular stimulation in producing speech sounds in an autistic child. *Occupational Therapy Journal of Research, 8*(3), 187–191.

Saks, E. R. (2013, January 27). Successful and schizophrenic. *New York Times*, p. 25.

Schaaf, R. C., Miller, L. J., Seawell, D., & O'Keefe, S. (2003). Children with disturbances in sensory processing: A pilot study examining the role of the parasympathetic nervous system. *American Journal of Occupational Therapy, 57*, 442–449.

Schneider, T., & Przewłocki, R. (2005). Behavioral alterations in rats prenatally exposed to valproic acid: Animal model of autism. *Neuropsychopharmacology, 30*, 80–89.

Schoen, S. A., Miller, L. J., Brett-Green, B. A., & Nielsen, D. M. (2009). Physiological and behavioral differences in sensory processing: A comparison of children with autism spectrum disorder and sensory modulation disorder. *Frontiers in Integrative Neuroscience, 3*(29), 1–11.

Schueli, H., Henn, V., & Brugger, P. (1999). Vestibular stimulation affects dichotic lexical decision performance. *Neuropsychologia, 37*(6), 653–659.

Siddiqi, S. U., Van Dyke, D. C., Donohoue, P., & McBrien, D. M. (1999). Premature sexual development in individuals with neurodevelopmental disabilities. *Developmental Medicine and Child Neurology, 41*(6), 392–395.

Silver, L. B. (1998). *The misunderstood child* (3rd ed.). New York: Three Rivers.

Soraya, L. (2013). The uncounted costs of sensory sensitivity. Asperger's Diary, *Psychology Today*. Retrieved from http://www.psychologytoday.com/blog/aspergers-diary/201301/the-uncounted-costs-sensory-sensitivity.

Stevens, L. J., Zentall, S. S., Abate, M. L., Kuczek, T., & Burgess, J. R. (1996). Omega-3 fatty acids in boys with behavior, learning, and health problems. *Physiology and Behavior, 59*(4–5), 915–920.

Stordy, J. (2000). *The LCP connection*. New York: Random House.

Thomas, A., Chess, S., & Birch, H. G. (1968). *Temperament and development*. New York: New York University Press.

Turecki, S. (2000). *The difficult child* (rev. ed.). New York: Bantam.

Volman, M. J. M., van Schendel, B. M., & Jongmans, M. J. (2006). Handwriting difficulties in primary school children: A search for underlying mechanisms. *American Journal of Occupational Therapy, 60*(4), 451–460.

Wakschlag, L. S., Choi, S. W., Carter, A. S., Hullsiek, H., Burns, J., McCarthy, K. . . . Briggs-Gowan, M. J. (2012). Defining the developmental parameters of temper loss in early childhood: Implications for developmental psychopathology. *Journal of Child Psychology and Psychiatry*. doi: 10.1111/j.1469-7610.2012.02595.

Warner, E., Cook, A., Westcott, A., & Koomar, J. (2011). *SMART: Sensory motor arousal regulation treatment*. Brookline, MA: Trauma Center at JRI.

Wilbarger, P. (1984). Planning an adequate sensory diet: Application of sensory processing theory during the first year of life. *Zero to Three. 10*, 7–12.

Williams, M. S., & Shellenberger, S. (1996). *How does your engine run? Leader's guide to the alert program for self regulation*. Albuquerque, NM: TherapyWorks.

Zero to Three. (2005). *Diagnostic classification of mental health and developmental disorders in infancy and early childhood* (rev. ed.). Washingon, DC: Author.

INDEX

Note: Italicized page locators indicate photos/illustrations.

overstimulation, 45, 79
oxybenzone, 164

pain, 8
    protecting child from, 94–98
    temperature and, 61
paper
    getting thoughts on, 235–36
    writing, 233
parasympathetic nervous system, SPD
    and differences in response, 56
parents, empowering strategies for,
    143–97
    daily life tasks, handling, 155–78
    dentists, doctors, and other
        professional visits, 185–90
    food issues, 178–83
    getting teachers on board around
        SPD issues, 247–48
    IEP meeting tips, 203–4
    meltdowns, handling, 154–55
    parties, holidays, and other group
        gatherings, 183–85
    preventive strategies, 152–54
    puberty, 193–97
    sensory problem vs. behavior
        problem, 146–52
    setting child up for success, 143–46
    sleep time, 190–93
parties, 183–85
passive hearing, 9
Pea Pod Student Calming Station, 98
Pediatools monkey, 113
pediatric ophthalmologists, 136, 224
peer pressure, 193
pencil grasp development, 228–30
pencil grips, molded, 231–32
persistence, 24
Peske, N., 61, 156
phonemes, 11
photosensitive students, lighting and,
    221–22
physical education class, 205
physical therapists (PTs), 126, 133–34,
    202
physical therapy, 132, 133
picky eaters, 178
Pilates, 119
pimple creams, 196
pink noise, 96

Play-Doh, 113, 185
playgrounds
    proprioceptive skills used in, 18
    vestibular sense and activity in, 19
play time, unstructured, at school,
    207–8
pollution, 88
posture
    bathing and, 158–59
    mealtime seating and, 171–72
    school and, 212–214
    toileting and, 167
    vestibular system and, 20
Potock, M., 182
pragmatic language, 11, 134
precocious puberty, 195
predictability and control, increasing,
    143–44
prematurity, 78, 86
problem eaters, tips for, 180–82
proprioceptive processing issues,
    61–64
    developing motor skills, 63
    factors to consider with, 19
    muscle tone, fatigue, and alterations
        in center of gravity, 63
    self-care and feeding problems, 64
    sensory seeking, 62
    space cadets, 62
    stimming and, 122
proprioceptive sense, 6, 17–19, 23
proprioceptive sensory system,
    vestibular system and, 20, 21
proprioceptive underreactivity,
    children with ASD and, 79
protective tactile input, 8
puberty, 193–97

quality of life, in sensory terms, 29
questionnaires, 101–2, 103–8, 127
quetiapine, 120

Raising a Sensory Smart Child (Biel
    and Peske), 61, 124, 249, 250
reading time, at school, 224–25
receptive language, 11, 68, 134
recess, school, 240–42
Rehabilitation Act of 1973, Section 504
    of, 200
repetitive behaviors, 55, 78, 119